Resource Management in Health and Social Care

Essential checklists

William Bryans

Radcliffe Publishing

Oxford ● San Francisco

Radcliffe Publishing Ltd
18 Marcham Road
Abingdon
Oxon OX14 1AA
United Kingdom

www.radcliffe-oxford.com
Electronic catalogue and worldwide online ordering facility.

British Library Cataloguing in Publication Data

A catalogue record for this book is available from the British Library.

ISBN 1 85775 627 4

Typeset by Aarontype Ltd, Easton, Bristol
Printed and bound by TJ International Ltd, Padstow, Cornwall

Contents

1120486

About the author

William Bryans is a specialist in health and social services business and financial management. The material in this book is based upon his wide managerial experience, his involvement with organisation and management development (including the implementation of the Management Education System through Open Learning (MESOL) project, developed by the Institute of Healthcare Management as a mode of entry to the profession), and various published articles and papers.

As a promoter of the workplace as a management college, as a university lecturer and as an external assessor he has always been acutely aware of the need for definitive literature which brings together practical business advice. As well as providing checklists of actions to take in specific circumstances, this book gives definitions, guidance, facts and advice about complex matters in clear unambiguous language. It also provides a framework that can be adapted to meet individual needs.

William is a Fellow of the Chartered Institute of Secretaries and Administrators (FCIS) and a Fellow of the Institute of Healthcare Management (FIHM).

About this book

Resource managers and frontline staff have to live with the fact that scarcity is a persistent and permanent economic phenomenon. It is a problem that will continue to be reflected in shortages of all types of essential resources.

When resource scarcity is mentioned it is natural to think only in terms of finance. But money may not be the only problem. Even when funds are available, there can be frustrating delays in obtaining priority items on the shopping list.

Some resources such as specialist clinical knowledge and experience take years to accumulate and others like commissioning new building stock may have similar time scales.

Resource Management in Health and Social Care provides a structured and integrated holistic approach to the rapidly developing health and social care environments that constantly test modern resource managers with daunting but often familiar challenges.

- Escalating patient and client expectations, and increasing demand especially in the older persons sector, are seldom matched with commensurate increases in resources.
- Whilst constantly improving techniques and technology facilitate better care and treatment, they often introduce unprecedented ethical and moral dilemmas.
- The general trend towards shorter stays at all levels of care has effectively precipitated the reduction in available beds with little appearance of creative thought applied to overcrowding problems in other parts of the care spectrum, for example the scandalously third-world care of patients waiting on trolleys in some Accident and Emergency Departments.
- This shorter stay trend also increases dependency at all levels.
- In order to cope, resource managers have to move beyond the confines of rations and budgets.
- In addition to their drive on waste, and reputation for good stewardship, they have to become competent in the political dimension where resource supply is regulated.
- They have to value and foster goodwill in all areas that have the potential to provide additional resources.

- Modern resource managers have to become skilled at developing appropriate partnerships.
- They must also constantly seek to reconcile patient and client expectations with available resources.

Managing in the climate of constant change

In addition to the pressures of meeting centrally imposed targets that may not be perceived locally as priorities, for example the annual ritual of balancing the books, etc., budget managers have a number of important external influences that they must take into consideration:

- clinical practice improvements, new technology and scientific discovery leading to a much broader spectrum of available treatments and care arrangements
- ageing population requiring increasing support and care
- increases in patient/relative/client expectation
- escalating patient/client numbers
- pressures arising from legal, ethical and moral judgements resulting from the application or otherwise of advances in the ability to care and treat conditions that had previously proved difficult or impossible
- unacceptable waiting times and length of waiting lists, including the length of time patients/clients have to spend in waiting areas
- near-zero financial growth climate
- continued alteration in the balance of care in favour of community, for example patients staying too long at an inappropriately high level of care in the acute sector and children possibly awaiting adoption in care homes in the child care sector.

Some of these influences, whilst requiring short-term investment, can have financially positive outcomes in the longer term, for example, the reduction in patient stays due to the constant introduction of new and less invasive techniques and the active precipitation from the highly acute sector into more appropriate and less expensive forms of care.

Rationale

Despite the multitude of official documentation and training programmes etc., managers at all levels and students continue to experience difficulties with the volatility altering costs.

One of the most confusing aspects of resource management is the fact that services must be maintained and indeed in some cases expanded, while attempts to reduce costs are proceeding in parallel. Already faced with apparently intractable problems, many managers suffer from a lack of complete comprehension.

In desperation, budget managers sometimes carry out inappropriate interventions that only add to their difficulties. Little wonder that budget managers may suffer from a sense of insecurity and isolation when they have to take those difficult decisions.

Resource Management in Health and Social Care should considerably diminish that isolation with its emphasis on the practical and 'what to do next'. It is packed with help and guidance that managers and students can apply to reduce real-time problems, thereby reducing the urgency.

The book covers every budget manager's dream – how to make significant savings from already over-stretched resources.

Naturally, there are no easy or quick solutions, but any manager or student working through this series of checklists, which are supported with short explanatory texts, appropriate diagrams and case studies, will discover an integrated approach which, applied over time, will get results.

Aims of the book

In addition to managers, prospective managers and students, there is a significant shortage of published material which bridges the gap between principles and practice, and which is readily accessible to the academic or the mature manager wanting to check out, update their own notes on, or dip into a particular budgetary aspect. Although this book will be useful to a much wider readership, there is a demand at post-graduate level both on the part of tutors wishing to update their knowledge and on the part of students who must develop their competence in this complex dimension.

The book will be of interest to all management levels and an accessible handbook for those who wish to review current arrangements or design a fresh approach to practical financial problems. The book should also provide contemporary reading for those engaged in general management.

- The material is firmly rooted in an ethos of maintaining or improving quality whilst making significant savings.
- Its application will therefore reduce mistakes and improve resource management by guiding managers through the maze of possible interventions.

- Readers will be assisted in tackling practical financial problems in a systematic and purposeful way.
- It will be a guide to organisations and useful to managers in all disciplines who endeavour to improve their own performance and the performance of their services in a climate of constant scarcity.

Focus of the material

The book concentrates on the day-to-day resource management problems and longer term implications that confront managers and frontline staff. In particular, the emphasis is on the constant need to make significant savings by increasing efficiency without detriment to the patient, client, relative or the general public.

Through the use of checklists, the book sets out clearly and concisely how to tackle various resource problems in an accessible way so that both the quality of care and the well-being of staff are enhanced rather than diminished. Where appropriate there will be cross-referencing.

The material is organised to assist managers and students to:

- cope with the perpetual dilemma of doing more with less
- help to diagnose existing problems
- take appropriate remedial action with obvious deficiencies
- apply tactical and strategic interventions at appropriate junctures
- positively participate in various processes
- assemble coherent cases for additional resources
- gain ready access to a wide spectrum of advice
- obtain guidance at critical moments
- improve their business, administrative and budgetary competences
- maintain a comprehensive source of reference.

Who will benefit from this book?

Although the book makes reference to the changing environment, the main thrust and emphasis are upon those factors that do not change:

> Physical resources, money and time are always scarce but there are many devices and incentives that help the manager to make the best possible use of that which is available.

The release of funds through improved efficiency means that the organisation can concentrate greater resources on those pressure issues, such as waiting-list reductions, that will greatly enhance *patient and client care.*

There is also greater scope to improve overall quality from initiatives that come from within the organisation and these will have a direct effect on *staff safety, security, morale and sense of well-being.*

Benefits will also accrue to *relatives and visitors,* who will experience better support and the prevalent sense of improved confidence.

Cost reductions either through greater through-put or savings, or both, *increase performance and provide a more secure basis for better accountability.*

Disclaimer

Whilst the case studies are based on real situations, all details, names etc., are pure fiction. Any resemblance or similarity to persons or places is completely coincidental.

Structure

In common with its predecessor, *Managing in Health and Social Care,* the main content and drive of this book are based around the checklist. Each chapter has:

- a purpose statement
- a list of main issues
- examples and illustrations, if appropriate
- hints and tips for managers wishing to improve competence
- copious checklists of practical steps for managers confronted with a specific problem
- numerous illustrative case studies.

The chapters are arranged as follows:

1 **Resources and sources of funding**
   Resources such as goods, expertise, estate, systems and equipment (GEESE) are scarce but with annual spending on health and social care estimated at over £85 billion, money is clearly the one resource that is not in short supply.

   - So why do managers have persistent funding difficulties?
   - Can managers gain better access to funds?
   - Do they really need more money to solve their problems?

2   **Balancing expectation with reality**
The connections that link expectation, resource availability, funding and service delivery are well recognised. Failure to meet reasonable expectations tends to result in resource wastage. In order to improve the situation an overview of the total picture is necessary. It is important to identify the problems and to take appropriate steps to reduce differences between expectation and reality.

3   **Resource deficits**
Shortages in the supply of money are not the sole cause of resource deficiencies. Certain key resources, for example highly qualified staff, can be scarce, particularly away from centres of excellence. Where there are shortages of key resources other than money, there will be an under-spending in terms of budget but prolonged deficiencies will prejudice the viability of a service.

4   **Quality, expectation and costs**
The complex means whereby the ever-increasing demand for a wide range of clinical options and different methodologies for the provision of social care is balanced with the reality of scarce resources is based upon basic economic principles. This is reflected in the strenuous efforts that are made to ensure equity (not always successfully) and effectiveness. Supply, demand, competition, cost and price have all been introduced to the health and social care vocabulary. This chapter gives an overview of how these principles are applied and provides guidance on how managers might respond.

5   **Managing within time limits**
In resource management, it is impossible to ignore the questions:

- Have we got the time to make adjustments or changes?
- Can we buy more time?
- How long will our resources last?
- What was accomplished in a given time?

Time is therefore both a measure of performance and a resource to be managed.

6   **Commissioning resources**
Appropriate and effective purchasing or commissioning of resources is crucial to quality and performance. However, because it is so specialised, often technical and frequently undertaken at a distance, managers have a tendency to leave the detail to the 'experts'. This can lead to mistakes, coupled with communication problems, that result in wasteful practices.

7   **Budgets and resources**
    Budgetary management is a critical measurement of resource performance
    and the need for appropriate intervention. It also gives an important
    insight into the affordability of the service provided and is a significant
    indicator of the need to reallocate resources. However, its effectiveness
    can be impaired because of flaws in organisational, structural or other
    management arrangements.

8   **Managing in the political dimension**
    The acquisition and consumption of resources are not in themselves
    objectives, but are rather the means by which objectives can be attained.
    However, a manager's ability to influence the main funding provider and
    to compensate for shortfalls by using suitable alternatives is an important
    asset in sustaining and developing services. In addition, managers must
    create an internal environment that attracts the right calibre of staff.

Often, when we think of resources, we mean money but although this is
an important aspect of resource management, money is simply the
medium that facilitates the purchase or commissioning of all those other
tangible and intangible items and skills required to make service provision happen.

   Therefore, the term '**resource managers**' applies not only to budget
holders but also to anyone who has responsibility for the consumption
of time, materials, equipment, estate, etc.

To Edith

1

Resources and sources of funding

Resources such as goods, expertise, estate, systems and equipment (GEESE) are scarce but with annual spending on health and social care estimated at over £85 billion money is clearly the one resource that is not in short supply.

- So why do managers have persistent funding difficulties?
- Can managers gain better access to funds?
- Do they really need more money to solve their problems?

The issues

In order to survive and develop services in a rapidly changing environment, modern health and social care managers must recognise and reconcile three fundamentally contradictory pressures that affect the way in which funds are used:

- constantly rising levels of expectation and demand for improvement
- significant increases in patient/client dependency and numbers
- a permanent climate of scarcity in the availability of physical resources.

Managers must also become intimate with the condition of their own environment and:

- assess the state of their current resources in terms of consumption, the degree of depreciation and the need for renewal or refreshment
- identify the sources of income that maintain and are available to develop their services.

Introduction

In the several, disparate and sometimes conflicting contexts of terms such as clinical governance, best value, and quality and excellence in resource management, many organisations in the health and social service spectrum continue to struggle with an integrated approach to the implementation of organisational excellence, performance measurement, process quality improvements, and physical and financial rectitude.

The debate about quality, expectation, the resource equation and excellence seems destined to run and run, but there can be little doubt that in attaining credible and measurable standards there is inevitably a heavy commitment to bureaucracy that some might argue would be better reallocated to the straight improvement of quality treatment and care that everyone seems to want. This introductory chapter provides an extensive overview of these complex relationships especially in the context of patient and service user focused services that inevitably consume resources.

Whilst political dimensions and relativity might differ, development and improvement in access to quality healthcare in return for realistic costs are recognisably familiar global problems. Unfortunately, none of these, nor many of the underlining factors for that matter, are fixed. Expectations tend to have an alarming tendency to escalate.

Obviously these characteristics create an unstable resource model because there is no evident counter-balancing measure(s) in the equation. Research, reform and increased bureaucracy can in these circumstances result in unsatisfactory quality, wasteful management costs and demoralising changes, which are in themselves uneconomic. If policy and decision makers, who are doubtless involved in complex choices, are either unaware or choose to ignore the equation that links quality to cost, then there will be dissatisfaction at all levels, including the consumer.

The role and performance of the manager

Budget managers' performance in a constant climate of change is greatly influenced by their ability to cope with increasing expectation and limited resource availability, and they have to be sure that the rate at which resources are consumed does not outstrip supply. Managers also have to know how to access more resources if they are needed.

It follows, therefore, that in order to succeed, managers must seek constant reassurance not only that their service has a future in the current situation but that they are well placed to renegotiate their resource position. For example, a service whose culture is firmly entrenched in maintaining overcapacity in order to cope with inappropriate forms of care for longer-stay patients will not be as favoured as a service where levels of care appropriate to the patient's/client's dependency are available at each stage.

Managers must ensure that their service is compatible with both internal and external pressures.

Case study

Despite the many changes and clinical developments mentioned, Smalltown Infirmary had managed to maintain its integrity as an acute hospital for the past three decades, providing good quality services to the local urban and the wider hinterland communities. Because its limited capacity restricted the number of specialist posts, it relied on the nearby St Bedeful in Bigtown to provide appropriate senior staff cover in times of pressure. But recently, the number of consultant vacancies in the infirmary rose alarmingly and the Director of Clinical Services has had to review the feasibility of continued acute care provision on the infirmary site.

Internal and external management environments are affected by those factors for change that are familiar to all health and social care managers, who must seek to either comply or influence opinion. The main sources of pressure are noted in the following checklist.

Checklist of main pressures for change

▼   Developments in clinical practice, new technology and scientific discovery leading to a much broader spectrum of available treatments and care arrangements.
▼   Ageing population requiring increasing support and care.
▼   A tendency to apply clinical safety criteria that require larger number of patient groupings to ensure economic provision of best practice (e.g. maternity services).
▼   Increases in patient/relative/client expectation, demand and patient/client numbers.
▼   Pressures arising from legal, ethical and moral judgements resulting from the application or otherwise of advances in the ability to care and treat conditions that had previously proved difficult or impossible.

▼ Unacceptable length of time waiting for appointments and length of waiting lists, including the length of time patients/clients have to spend in waiting areas.
▼ Near-zero financial growth climate.
▼ Need to further reduce costs, make savings and increase income.
▼ Continued alteration in the balance of care in favour of community (e.g. continuing development of less invasive surgical techniques that permit increases in day surgery and earlier discharge).
▼ Innovative remedies for intractable problems that inhibit the best use of appropriate beds or other spaces at critical points in the delivery of care and/or treatment to clients and patients. For convenience, these pressures are generally divided into three groups:

  – the escalation in both demand and expectation
  – the flow of funding and other resources into the health and social care system.

▼ The utility, efficiency and effectiveness that are manifested by the system in producing the most efficacious management, care and treatment of the disorders presented.

This dynamic climatic arrangement is illustrated in Figure 1.1.

In this bewildering climate, modern managers are under constant and increasing pressure to improve their services. Paradoxically, medicine, science and technology have provided both the prospect of going some way towards achieving those improvements and at the same time, the means to frustrate those aims.

To a large extent, this anomaly is caused by the difficulty in creating the necessary degree of flexibility in finance that would facilitate more mobility in the way more physically permanent resources such as buildings and, to a lesser extent, skilled resources are managed.

Bridging the gap(s) in resource provision

Deviations between the amount of resources available and the established need are regular occurrences. Usually, but not always, the deviation is characterised by a supply shortfall. In this situation, managers at all levels often consider the budget reductions first, but augmenting resources from

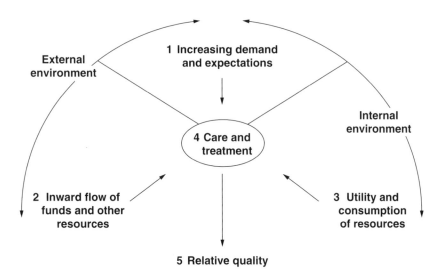

Figure 1.1   Climate pressures and the environment.*

*Notes
1   *Escalating pressure* on service commissioning and provision arises from continued developments and discovery in care and treatment, higher expectation of improvements and the inherent occurrence of ethical and moral dilemmas.
2   *The inward flow of funds and other resources* is a limiting factor upon capability and capacity of the existing service provision. The situation has prospects of improvement where the service conforms with a desire to influence or conform with expectation. Accordingly, managers have to create an awareness of and learn to manage this aspect of their external environment.
3   *Utility and consumption of resources.* Within their internal environment, managers must work tirelessly to find the most effective ways that resources can be deployed and used.
4   *Care and treatment.* Managers have to ensure that the *appropriate* level of care and treatment commensurate with available resources is provided. This means that they must monitor constantly, review and renegotiate levels of resource provision according to need.
5   *Relative quality.* This will be the perceived outcome and results from the management response to the many pressures that are implicit in service commissioning and provision. It is relative in terms of a number of complex factors such as expectation, previous experience, cultural norms, education and individual requirements.

other sources can be an equally successful strategy and is certainly one that, even if not wholly a solution, should be implemented in parallel with a savings plan.

When we think of income sources, the taxpayer immediately comes to mind as the main contributor to both locally and nationally provided health and social care. However, we rely heavily upon a very large private sector to undertake those risky and time-consuming aspects of research, development and production of specialist material resources such as drugs and equipment.

A section of the private sector also provides private care to a variety of patients/clients thus alleviating pressure on the main provider. In addition there are numerous examples of voluntary or charitable services that give invaluable help at crucial and often sensitive junctures in the care–treatment continuum.

In the well-developed budgetary environment therefore, successful managers at all levels take care to ensure that they manage their internal environment. But they are also perceived to pay particular attention to all aspects of their external environment where major help, goodwill, general support and, most importantly, extra resources can be mobilised for the benefit of the services they provide.

This approach to the external environment is best developed as part of an overall organisational culture in which protocols and methodologies form a flexible framework in which managers can operate. Unless there are inherent contractual, moral obligations or ethical considerations, this framework should not be an inhibiting factor that limits individual managers undertaking normal day-to-day communications with interested external parties.

Influencing external elements

Taxpayers are the main source of income for both health and social care. Managers must fully comprehend how their funds can be increased and where appropriate, why there appears to be a shortfall. These will be areas for possible consultation, negotiation and re-negotiation, lobbying, media coverage and submitting or resubmitting cases (the political dimension). It follows that managers have to become competent in dealing effectively with this important funding source. We shall therefore be returning to this crucial feature of budgetary and resource management, but first it is important to create an awareness of the many other sources of income and support that are available.

In this context, managers have to appreciate the value of the many external influences that can benefit services by augmenting overstretched resources in tangible or perhaps less obvious ways. Conversely, it is equally important to be alert to those influences which, because of other considerations, may not be welcome. We have to be prepared for both situations and know how to deal with them.

The checklist below covers most of those areas where goodwill can be fostered and additional complementary resources mobilised.

Checklist of possible sources of complementary or additional resources

▼ *Private enterprise.* This covers a wide spectrum of interest from those who already supply goods and services to the organisation through to those enterprises that are coterminous in that they share common ground or goals. Commercial organisations, both large and small, are often willing to offer physical help or sponsorship deals in return for a modest gain, for example advertising. Care has to be taken, however, that there is no conflict of interest either on an ethical basis (e.g. tobacco products) or in conferring an unfair commercial advantage to a trader. A checklist of relevant considerations is included at the end of the chapter.

▼ *Gifts and endowments.* Money and physical resources can flow from this valuable source, but managers who are involved in advice or encouragement of donors need to be aware of the pitfalls that can result from an inappropriate offer. Suggested criteria that might be used to judge the potential benefits of a proposal are listed at the end of the chapter.

▼ *Voluntary workers.* Most health and social care organisations derive considerable benefit from the voluntary worker cadre. Many examples come to mind ranging from the person who provides a tuck-shop service and the voluntary driver, to the hospital or care facility visitor who provides company and companionship to those most in need. Whilst it is vitally important to encourage and develop all these individual contributions, it is also critical that organisations have policy guidelines that both limit and at the same time direct activity to areas where voluntary work is acceptable and appropriate. Where areas of work are sensitive or where there may be a potential risk, some health and social care organisations strictly regulate voluntary workers, provide them with honorary contracts and clearly identify them in order to secure a safe environment.

▼ *Local support groups and charitable organisations.* Although relations with the majority of patients, clients and relatives may be transient, there are nevertheless a substantial number who are sensitive both to the scarcity of resources in a particular area and to the benefits inherent in new developments in care and treatment. This fund of goodwill is frequently mobilised around specific projects, and health and social care organisations and their staff should be constantly alert to the potential benefits that can be derived from these coordinated efforts. Outright refusal of help is bad for morale and bad for public relations. Where there is a problem with a proposal, for example if the suggestion would lead to unreasonably high costs to the organisation immediately or at a later date, strenuous efforts should be made as early as possible to advise and direct efforts towards fruitful developments. It is important, therefore, to identify and encourage all those who are prepared to make a coordinated effort to enhance an organisation's capability and to work with them in securing funding that will be mutually beneficial. This is dealt with in more detail in the section on taxpayer funding below (*see* page 10).

▼   *National charities*. Links and relationships with relevant national charities that are dedicated to the improvement in the state of care or knowledge of particular groups are desirable. During this process, it may be discovered that a particular gap in service provision can be closed by the pooling of resources, perhaps even on a permanent basis, for example with the provision and/or the equipping of a new building.

▼   *Partnerships*. In order to make the best possible use of resources and to ensure the provision of a seamless and uninterrupted service, the government is keen to promote partnerships with others in the public sector, particularly with social services in respect of care of the elderly. It is interesting to note that in addition to examples of partnerships on mainland UK, in Northern Ireland health and personal social services have been commissioned and delivered by single commissioner/provider-integrated arrangements since 1973. Checklists relating to partnerships are dealt with in Chapter 8. However, it is important to note that similar benefits in respect of sharing resources can often be achieved through the use of other forms of partnership in all the sectors mentioned above.

▼   *Savings programmes*. The need for managers to make savings or create a surplus is a naturally occurring, if grossly understated, management function. There are four main reasons for its existence:

– to reduce the prevalence of waste, fraud, negligence, etc.
– to bridge the funding gap forecast
– to provide a contingency from which managers may seek to develop their services
– a combination of two or all three of the above – probably the most likely reason.

The creation of flexibility by releasing funds through savings is difficult because money is locked into health and social care systems and culture in such a way that its redirection for other, and perhaps more beneficial purposes, becomes a daunting task. Before embarking upon a savings programme, managers must value, appreciate and understand the extent and limits of their sources of income. They have to know the exact purpose of the money they have received or are about to receive: they will not be permitted to save in approved growth areas.

Other theoretically possible alternative funding arrangements

Over the decades, many ideas have been floated for the creation of increased funding. These are mainly based upon two considerations. First, there is the notion that at local level, in concert with greater autonomy, there should be a commensurate facility to increase or improve the funding capability. This notion has already been carried into practice to a certain extent through the limited power to raise capital funds.

The second consideration rests upon the idea that patients and clients should pay for some or all of those services that are part of everyday life, mainly hotel services. However, in order to preserve a measure of fairness, a nightmare bureaucracy would have to be created. In the case of social care, particularly residential care, and in the case of pensioners going into hospital for lengthy periods of time, recipients already have to pay, so there are some precedents. However, in recent times the idea of the elderly paying for that which can be termed 'nursing care' has been successfully challenged.

Below is a short checklist of some of the ideas that have been put forward as likely sources of additional income.

Checklist of ideas for alternative funding

▼ *Local taxation.* On the surface this seems to be a relatively simple and reasonably sensible suggestion. Indeed, in the case of social care there is an obvious connection (except in Northern Ireland where health and social care is an integrated package). But in the case of healthcare, it fails on the principle that links taxation to representation. This is because there is no clear local link between the taxpayer and trusts. In addition, at local level there is already a high dependency on government grants and where a variation or significant change occurs, the local taxpayer generally bears the deficiency. In some parts of the UK, this has recently caused considerable outrage and it is difficult to see how a further burden would be made acceptable.

▼ *Reimbursement of damages, etc.* There is a wide spectrum of injuries that result in the payment of damages. In the case of road accidents, health trusts are entitled to their appropriate share of the settlement. However, other injuries, including those connected with sporting activities, are the subject of debate. In addition, diseases that have occurred through deliberate negligence on the part of either the patient or a third party are being scrutinised to see whether costs arising from their care and treatment could be retrieved from sources other than the public purse. Such proposals would be difficult to implement both because of the legalistic aspects inherent in the burden of proof and because of the social implications that might arise from deterring patients from seeking timely and effective help.

▼ *Paying for housekeeping.* A surprising 20% of gross expenditure is allocated to catering, cleaning, portering, linen and other related services. The argument that favours patients having to make a contribution to these services is based on the notion that a significant portion of these would be costs normally incurred by the patient. However, unless proposed charges are pitched at a realistic level, the cost of recovery might turn out to be uneconomic.

▼ *Voluntary contributions.* This can be easily confused with the many voluntary contributions that grateful patients, relatives and others make to gift and endowment funds. In essence there would be no distinction except that the gift or money would go directly into special accounts in public funds for the uses specified. As with gift and endowment funds, the main problems arise from the complexity and age of the funds created and it is generally thought that it is better to keep the two aspects separate.

Taxpayer funding

In the case of local authority provision of services such as personal social care, local community charges only account for around 25% of expenditure. Apart from contributions from service users, the rest is found mainly from government grants.

Thus, if this main source of income is varied in order to maintain services at the same level, the effect on the local taxpayer will triple in its impact. When this is to the local taxpayer's significant disadvantage, then there is a natural adverse reaction.

However, downward pressure of increased expectation due to care in the community initiatives and contracting-out services, coupled with careful budgeting, often results in service recipients feeling that the amount of time allocated to their needs is inadequate, for example the well-publicised limitation on home help and carer provision.

In the case of the NHS, taxpayer funding is considerably further removed from the actual source of funds (i.e. the taxpayer). The result is that the taxpayer, despite a veneer of consultative and watchdog processes, has virtually no input into how services are to be structured and provided. At the taxpayer level the complex of commissioner/provider contractual and other arrangements must appear unduly bureaucratic.

Indeed, it might be that there are some within the service who might be confused as to how the system really works and if they did know, they might be further surprised that it actually works at all. All this and other relevant issues such as the proposed system of national tariffs will be discussed in more detail in succeeding chapters.

Key action points

In order to cope with increasing and conflicting pressures in a climate of constant change, health and social care managers have to:

▼ indentify the higher expectations of improvements in health and social care provision that apply to their specialist area
▼ forecast or otherwise specify increases or decreases in patient/client dependency and numbers
▼ create an awareness of the commensurate escalation in the rate at which resources are consumed
▼ manage within a strict code of efficiency and effectiveness
▼ relate the permanent state of physical resource scarcity to their specific circumstances, e.g. manpower shortages
▼ be prepared to look at alternative means to bridge gaps in the funding process
▼ make a general action plan that covers the particular situation.

Case study

At County Hall in Bigtown, the Director of Social Services, despite ever more pressing demands from an increasingly elderly population, has had to face another year of reduced spending. This means cuts (although she never uses that word) in home help provision and general community care. In addition there are bound to be more problems from a fining system that will impose sanctions on social services that are slow to act in finding places for people who were inappropriately placed in the acute hospital system.

Tips from the front office

▼ Taxpayers/patients/clients are in some form the paymasters of health and social care.
▼ Managers and other professionals must therefore be sensitive to their needs and expectations.
▼ Management of the political dimension has to be the result of a balanced approach to holistic resource management.

2

Balancing expectation with reality

The connections that link expectation, resource availability, funding and service delivery are well recognised. Failure to meet reasonable expectations tends to result in resource wastage. In order to improve the situation an overview of the total picture is necessary. It is important to identify the problems and to take appropriate steps to reduce differences between expectation and reality.

The issues

At every level, both inside and outside the health or social care organisation, increased or deliberately raised expectations of service improvements will constantly exceed the reality. A balance must therefore be struck between expectation, competing priorities and the reality of scarcity. This chapter gives a broad indication of what to look for and where to look for it. The main headings are:

- Historical and future context – managers need to have a sense of traditional expectation before they can plan for the future
- Expectation – as a mathematical function of previous experience
- Perceived expectation – in professional areas as it affects patients/clients
- Broad indicators and measures that may be taken to reduce dissonance
- Commissioner/provider expectations.

Introduction

The complex means whereby we harmonise the ever-increasing demand for a wide range of clinical options with the reality of scarce resources is the result of an inevitable balance between competing priorities. But whether we can deliver devices that will reduce the dissonance so frequently experienced when either allocating or analysing the distribution of wealth throughout the NHS is subject to constant debate and analysis.

Retrospectively, whilst the range and scope of treatment options spiral upwards, it becomes ever easier to criticise decisions on resource investment. Even those decisions that might at the time have appeared trivial can lead to bitter acrimony. It is therefore a natural response to hedge the decision-making process with sometimes piecemeal safeguards. Because of the usual time constraints on spending, these can, and often do, result in administrative stagnation and the loss of an opportunity.

However, the fact that prevalence of scarcity at all levels is a management axiom does not compensate for increasing demand and expectation. In health and social care, resource shortages dominate both service provision and resource management. And scarcity pervades every aspect ranging from that vague public expectation through the resource commissioning processes, to the patient/client/relative perception of the final delivery of a 'quality'-assured service.

One of the consequences is that at every level, increased or deliberately raised expectations of a service will constantly exceed the reality. Where possible, managers must take steps to ensure that so-called supercharged expectations are put in optimistic perspective. They must also be sure that shortages are managed in such a way that the gap between expectation and provision is small. However, it often happens that resources may become available to meet the expectation of a particular development and managers have to be prepared for this eventuality.

Deficiencies in the quality of life of the population served are apparent in population profiles. These statistics are concerned mainly with the age structure, birth rates, death and accidental incident statistics, and the relative material poverty of different sectors of the population. Health and social service managers recognise the relevance of these factors to the problems that they have to deal with. For example, on a national level:

- life expectancy at birth is 74 for men and 79 for women
- the birth rate is about 13 per 1000
- infant deaths in a population of 59 million are 5000
- deaths under 1 year per 1000 live births are 6
- total death rate per 1000 is 10.7.

If the cost per capita was allowed to rise to £1,500 in 2004/05, we might expect the distribution of that cost to be as shown in Table 2.1.

Table 2.1 Estimate of the cost of health and personal social services per head of population served

Cost per capita

Detail	Cost
Hospital and related services	712
Community health services	124
Family practitioner services	356
Personal social services	228
Management costs	80
Total	£1,500

In order to gain an idea of deficiencies within a particular area, it is necessary to take account of both the current situation and rapidly emerging priorities. This means realistically considering:

- external environmental influences, which include expectation of patients, clients, relatives and the general public
- reality of the internal environment, especially in the context of resource management
- performance in the provision of appropriate care and treatment.

Reflection upon commercial practice

It has been suggested that a number of quality dimensions can be applied to the healthcare environment. They are accessibility, equity, relevance to need, acceptability, efficiency and effectiveness. Many authorities have adopted and adapted these dimensions as key components of their own quality initiatives. Indeed they are familiar reading to those who spend time perusing the volumes of commissioning documentation. It is vitally important to note that although these noble aspirations are fundamental headline material, they are all on the same side of the quality equation. As has already been demonstrated, accessibility and equity do not always equal efficiency and effectiveness. A balance must be struck as to the degree and emphasis to be given to each dimension. With these reservations in mind, it is possible to evaluate broadly the significance of quality statements as a means of influencing the external environment.

Checklist of aspects of health and social care quality culture

Following through the path described for prospective customers above, it is possible to arrive at a checklist which will provide a broad outline of the culture of quality in a health or social care environment:

▼ *Directories/catalogues*. It is often thought that reference points to social- and healthcare are limited in interest to clients and patients, but this ignores the importance of information to other interested parties such as suppliers, recruitment agencies and schools, and communities with parallel concerns (e.g. business, professional, pastoral, local, etc.). Readable structured material providing initial access, help and guidance to service provision is an essential aspect of accessibility to who does what, where and when. GP practice guides are good examples. It is, however, important to update this material and check its relevance as a frequent quality audit task. This is a broad test of accessibility.

▼ *Market connection*. This is a little-understood marketing phenomenon that predates the internal market. It is a term that describes the established referral patterns experienced by most health and social care professionals. Its importance therefore transcends internal market requirements. Any quality evaluation must take account of the way health and social care referrals are received and accepted, together with an examination of how professionals in the system value or wish to influence these patterns. This is a broad test for a number of dimensions: accessibility, acceptability and relevance.

▼ *Reputation*. This is a key factor to all aspects of quality. 'A good name is better than precious ointment' is a quotation from the book of Ecclesiastes. The comparison is both appropriate and relevant in modern times. A reputation built upon a successful quality service must be the focus of patient/client care. It is central to the maintenance of the market connection. When a patient/client makes an appointment to see a particular professional, they expect that arrangement to be honoured – the very act of choice endows the relevant professional with the authority to deal with the problem presented. It is therefore counterproductive to deny access to the chosen professional without giving a proper explanation. This will test retrospective effectiveness and the emphasis on relevance to need.

▼ *Communication*. As in the commercial world, a patient/client does not expect to have to queue or otherwise stand in line. They want to feel that the professional is listening carefully and comprehending their problem, and that all the relevant details are being noted. This will test accessibility, relevance to need and efficiency.

▼ *Clear options.* Patients/clients expect to be told the truth and they need to hear the dangers and hazards inherent in the various options available in the remedies for their conditions – what is likely to happen to them, what precautions will be taken for their safety and the availability of treatment. This will test equity.

▼ *Agreement.* In arriving at a decision, patients/clients need time to consider. There must be evidence of a clear consensus on the proposed approach. This will be a test of acceptability.

▼ *Transaction.* Although an actual consideration is not a direct part of the transaction, there is nevertheless a cost in terms of the quality of opportunity for improvements. All parties to the agreement to the proposed treatment regime must be made aware of this factor. A broad evaluation will test efficiency and effectiveness.

▼ *Aftercare.* A statement of the need for adequate aftercare or follow-up system seems to be listing the obvious but sadly, too often, the exit advice to a patient or client is to '... *do this or take that* ...'. The fact that they do not turn up again for a further consultation or treatment is taken as a satisfactory outcome. A famous legal quotation seems appropriate – '... quiescence is not acquiescence ...'. Success needs more assurance than silence. Attitudes to this aspect will test effectiveness.

▼ *Complaints.* A complaints procedure, conciliation, analysis of complaints received and the steps taken to ensure that a particular set of circumstances is avoided in future are essential in quality development. This tests both efficiency and effectiveness.

▼ *Rectification.* Where a mistake has occurred, it is important to have a plan which deals adequately with all aspects of the occurrence, including staff support, so that its nature and incidence are properly understood and appropriate remedies applied. The existence of such a scheme tests efficiency and effectiveness.

A general overview is illustrated in Figure 2.1.

Resource considerations, performance levels and the requirements of the external environment, as represented mainly by the income likely to flow across the boundaries, are reconciled with emphasis on quality and the desired balance of care. This task is undertaken through a combination of financial, statistical and factual analyses.

Although the patient/client/relative/public expectation is of primary concern, expectation of an improved condition is manifested at every level

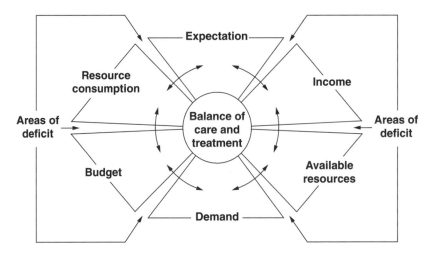

Figure 2.1   Overview of deficiencies in health and social care.

in health and social care organisations. Thus the management, staff, staff associations, suppliers and contractors all have expectations that often exceed reality. These in turn have an overall effect that influences perceived deficiencies at all the main intersections. Below is a checklist of the main interrelationships where deficits occur.

Checklist of interrelationships where deficits tend to occur

▼   *Patient/client/relative expectation − income provided.* The amount of funding provided for a service seldom reflects its increasingly ambitious public expectations. This is often exaggerated by premature announcements of 'discoveries' in more beneficial care and treatment.

▼   *Income − resource availability.* Although there may be sufficient funds in a system, the physical resources and skills needed may not be available, for example the acute shortages in nursing and other key staff.

▼   *Patient/client/relative   expectation − care   and   treatment − demand.* Through interaction with the care and treatment regime, the actual demand may not be as great as the expectation.

▼   *Income − budgets.* The total amount of income should equal the total amount in the budget. However, sometimes monies are set aside for contingencies or are otherwise earmarked for specific purposes and managers have to keep these amounts under close review so that maximum benefit is achieved.

▼   *Budgets – resource consumption – care and treatment.* The overall objectives in budget and resource management are to ensure that resource consumption does not exceed the budget and that the proper level and quality of care and treatment are maintained. This means a constant drive on wasteful practices and continuous monitoring of the quality and quantity of care and treatment.

▼   *Resource consumption – care and treatment – expectation.* Through the interaction of patients/clients/relatives/public with care and treatment provision as dictated by effective use of resources, a gradual revision of expectation will take place.

Historical and future context

There is little chance of long-term success in resource management where there is a critical mass of negative external factors. For example:

•   If government policy favours community-based initiatives for certain treatments or care, then there is little chance of a development that is not amenable to that kind of approach (i.e. creating a new demand for longer-term care or treatment).

•   Similarly, if departmental or commissioner preference directs funding towards other schemes, managers whose services are not so favoured must consider their options as to how their services can be made to fit the established criteria or how they can be persuasive about the efficiency and effectiveness of their form of care and treatment.

•   In the end, managers may need to come to terms with the need for change.

However this does not mean that because external opinion is against a particular proposal, managers must abandon a cherished scheme; instead they should seek to create an external climate in which their proposals will have a better chance. This aspect will be explored in more detail in Chapter 4.

It is important to provide a feel for the traditions of service that have so far influenced service development and to create an historical profile. The checklist below covers the main points to bear in mind.

Checklist of historical and current context for improvement

▼   Although the original purpose may be out of date, for example a sanatorium for TB, details provide an interesting and sometimes, in the case of core values, important background.

▼ Note the date when the service or building was founded.
▼ Trace any relevant milestone and changes that have occurred along the way.
▼ The location and accessibility of the service to the catchment, resident, patch or referred population should also be noted.
▼ Follow this with detailed descriptions of current service provision, growths in volume of care and treatments, size of budget, etc.
▼ Proposals for any developments must take account of the following factors:

  – expected patient/client volumes in the area for development, together with forecasted effects on other aspects
  – additional resources required
  – note whether the proposals are compatible with an alteration in the balance of care in favour of shorter stays in hospital/residential care
  – consider the impacts on resource management of increased dependency in both residual hospital and community-based populations
  – consequent increased burden on existing community services, for example the impact of earlier discharge policies.

Case study

The Director of Clinical Services at Smalltown Infirmary was concerned that the new laminar-flow twin theatres had so far failed to encourage the decentralisation of orthopaedics from the regional centre of excellence, located sixty miles plus from the general Smalltown hinterland. The new theatres were more accessible for the increasingly older rural population and would have taken up much of the spare surgical division beds made vacant by the increases in keyhole techniques. Falling inpatient numbers were a threat to viability.

Expectation

As stated earlier, the possession of an expectation in this context is not restricted to the patient/client/relative/public group but has important connotations for resource managers over a wide spectrum of their management functions. Interestingly, the 'expector' characteristics tend to be common to all aspects. Below is a general statement of this situation.

> **Expectation at a particular time is equal to a function of the know-ledge and experience already gained by the expector.**

This can be written in the form of an equation

$$E_t = f(K_{t-1})$$

where E is current expectation at a time t and K is knowledge or previous experience at a time just before t.

In addition, knowledge or previous experience is a composite and complex notion that is attained as a result of a number of key influences. These are included in the checklist below.

Checklist of key influences on experience

▼ The *education and capability* to fully appreciate the situation are of obvious importance, but in Western society, because it may be interpreted as patronising, it is not for practitioners to judge the degree of competence exhibited by a person. Where a clash of cultures exists between the practitioner and the patient/client/relative group, then problems may occur that have to be addressed through adequate training and development programmes. This aspect cannot be left unattended in the hope that time alone will improve matters.

▼ *Gender* has always been a key consideration both in terms of physical requirements and as far as segregation is concerned.

▼ Consideration of the *emotional state* is relevant to anyone facing a personal crisis. Their perception will focus on their main concern and this may exclude all other salient points. However in retrospect, they will recall the degree of sensitivity with which their problem was attended.

▼ The overall state of health and welfare services as represented by *cultural norms* will determine a basic attitude and anticipation. Where no health or social services exist, the population may expect none.

▼ *Social status or position in society* should not be a consideration, except at times when a particular person's special function should be maintained; for instance, leaders and key workers in a time of national or local crisis are needed to provide continuity.

▼ The function or economic role that a person performs means that their requirements differ, for example an athlete has different *job requirements* in terms of fitness to those of a person in a more sedentary occupation.

▼ The *increasing rate of clinical development* and growing sophistication in care and treatment, including less intrusive techniques, are well publicised and have a degree of impact on the expectations of patients and clients.

▼ *New technology* also enhances the expected benefits at all levels, although the mixed reception to the recent government initiative to improve the technology available to clinical services is indicative of the fear or lack of trust with which many still view 'progress' in this sector.

▼ With the increases in scientific and clinical discoveries, expectors at all levels in health and social care organisations are often drawn into *moral and ethical issues* which were not considerations a few years ago. Similarly, today's pressures produce a depressing and some-times emotionally charged perception of health service managers caught in a web of jargon, codes of practice and convention which actually diminishes the capacity to appreciate that changes to suit the requirements of the moment may rapidly become out of date. Today's acceptable practice may be considered barbaric tomorrow. Thus expectations in this respect have to be constantly reviewed to see whether they conform to requirements.

Case study

Mr H O'Condriac had difficulty following what the hospital doctor was saying to him. So he smiled, nodded and agreed at junctures in the con-versation when the doctor looked as though he expected him to be positive. And if Mr O'Condriac thought a negative response was appropriate, then he made sure he complied because he didn't want to annoy the doctor.

At this juncture, neither the doctor nor the patient was aware of any differences in their perception of how the consultation had progressed.

Perceived expectation

The realisation of perceived expectation will affect the way in which patients and clients react to a proposed regime. This can have either a positive or a negative outcome depending on the starting point. It is vitally important that the health and social care professional constantly bears in mind the dread with which a patient or client might present a problem to them.

Similarly if patients and clients feel that they have been made unduly uncomfortable during the course of their treatment or that they have experienced degrading or painful treatment, they may not complain, but they may not come back.

In resource management terms, where a patient or client fails to comply with a prescribed regimen, valuable resources will have been wasted and will be wasted in the future because of the potentially deteriorating condition.

This is one of the main reasons for such an emphasis on expectation in this context. In popular culture, the checklist that follows gives an indication of the key boxes that most people want to tick in order to meet their best expectations. Although it is couched in patient/client terminology, it is equally applicable to any health and social care relationship.

Checklist of key expectations and perceptions

▼ *Reputation.* 'A good name is better than precious ointment' Ecclesiastes, 7.1. Despite much-publicised league tables, most patients follow established referral patterns and rely on the health organisation to provide reputable care and treatment. Although there may not be the same choices, roughly the same criteria apply to social care provision. It is vitally important that health and social care organisations take steps to analyse exactly what their reputation is based on and to devise means to protect and enhance their situation.

▼ *Waiting lists.* The management of waiting lists consumes resources. This potentially diminishes the efficacy of care and treatment whilst at the same time increasing the potential cost. In problematic situations, where a loss of time may potentially cause a deterioration, most people should reasonably expect not have to wait overlong for an appointment. More than a few weeks would be too long to wait to see a solicitor or an accountant, so it's too long for other purposes.

▼ *Waiting times.* After the first appointment, it is reasonable to expect treatment to begin forthwith. This would be compatible with a reduction in potential waste. Also in this context, when an appointment has been made, patients and clients have a right to be seen on time at the appointed time.

▼ *Professionalism.* Failure to conform to professional standards can result in losses due to negligence, or worse. Patients/clients have a reasonable expectation to be received and treated appropriately.

This usually means acting in accordance with an established and recognised code of practice.

▼ *Assurance/reality.* This important aspect is often overlooked because it is difficult to regulate. In the current blame/claim climate, clinicians and other professionals, in their eagerness to avoid litigation, often leave patients and clients with more to worry about than is strictly necessary. Whilst the reality of the situation is important, someone who is already deeply concerned at the possible seriousness of their problem needs reassurance if time and effort are to be saved.

▼ *Security and safety.* Entry into the health and social care systems implies security and safety. Measures to save resources by taking risks in these areas are counterproductive and breaches in basic standards destroy trust.

▼ *Continuity of care and treatment.* Patients/clients expect a continuity of care. If this cannot be guaranteed (the key worker principle), resources have been wasted and expectations are unfulfilled.

Case study

Mr H O'Condriac was admitted to St Bedeful Hospital for further investigations. The side ward was overcrowded (seven beds where there should have been four) and the fire doors were obstructed. But the nursing staff, although clearly at breaking point, were always pleasant to him and nothing seemed to be too much trouble. Thinking that he might help prevent an outbreak of food poisoning, he mentioned the fact that dirty cutlery had been received at several mealtimes and other patients said they had had a similar experience. Eventually the quality assurance manager arrived to interview him and informed Mr H O'Condriac that the catering contractor was independent and therefore outside the scope of the quality inspectorate. If Mr O'Condriac wished to take the matter further, he would have to complete a questionnaire. Mr O'Condriac declined.

Checklist of anecdotal instances of patient/client dissonance

▼ No car parking spaces are left for disabled people.
▼ Negative reception such as 'You're lucky to be seen at all ...'
▼ Inappropriate office notices such as 'You don't have to be mad ...'
▼ Consultants never appear, even though they are supposed to be in charge of clinics.

▼ Patients' notes are not available or incorrect ones have been delivered.

▼ Perception of chaos at ward or clinic level.

▼ Lack of privacy to discuss intimate details.

▼ Obvious safety hazards like blocked fire exits.

▼ Critical or patronising attitude from the doctor.

▼ No apparent effort made to comprehend or take on board peripheral information from the patient, for example telling the doctor about a separate disease or discomfort.

▼ Over cautious consultation by junior doctor who may exhibit lack of knowledge.

▼ Uncomfortable/painful/undignified examination.

▼ Unnecessary expression of concern about likely seriousness of disease.

▼ 'Best to be sure ...' – onward referrals for further tests or consultations.

▼ Disclaimer notices in cubicles in circumstances when the patient already feels vulnerable and anxious.

Commissioner/provider expectations

Within health and social care organisations, and between them, expectation is a key motivating factor for staff. It is a fundamental management principle that managers and commissioners share the common goal of achieving as much return as possible for investment or purchases.

This creates downward pressure upon junior staff and providers to deliver more. If this pressure is perceived in consistently negative terms, it can be quietly devastating for both morale and service delivery. In extreme cases, the following rule comes into play.

Where commissioners and managers manifest an abiding conviction that providers and junior managers have more resources than they require, providers and junior managers will overcompensate by demanding more than they require.

Commissioners and managers rightly want more quality activity for less money (QUALM). However, we have to avoid the growth of a subculture in providers and junior managers that encourages waste by creating demands for more than is needed (DEMN). It is not sensible to leave these matters unresolved.

Case study

Incredibly, until recently, managers in St Bedeful Hospital permitted repeat and other stock requisitions to be completed by junior staff. When there were insufficient supplies in store to keep everyone happy, resolution of the dilemma was undertaken by the lowest common denominator, the store-keeper (not to diminish the role of storekeepers). For years he had applied a rough rationing technique until stocks were replenished, but when he retired nobody knew his secret.

Expectation of government funding

As far as the NHS is concerned, the main source of funds is through government and this structure is illustrated in Figure 2.2. From this it will be observed that, unlike social care provision where the taxpayer/client is near to the point of delivery, the taxpayer/patient has little or no political impact on how healthcare is provided.

Key action points

In order to cope with increasing and conflicting pressures in a climate of constant change, health and social care managers have to take into account:

▼ the creation of a sense of traditional expectation before they can plan for the future
▼ expectation as a mathematical function of previous experience
▼ perceived expectation in professional areas as it affects patients/clients
▼ broad indicators and measures that may be taken to reduce dissonance
▼ commissioner/provider expectations.

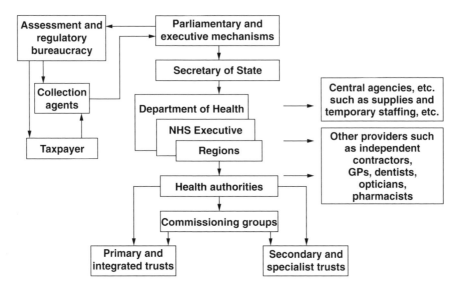

Figure 2.2   NHS funding – simplified overview.*

* Notes
- The diagram shows some of the levels of bureaucracy, but does not include functions such as the treasury, parliamentary and external scrutiny arrangements or the details of the government in each of the UK nations, excluding England.
- Although the functions in organisations including and below the Department of Health become more and more locally specific, the staffing, departmental representation and structure tend to be similar. For example, there will be finance and human resources departments at every level. As far as the flow of funds is concerned, this can be facilitating. On the other hand, it can also reduce the speed with which decisions are taken and executed.
- When taxpayers, who ultimately fund the NHS by one device or another, require care and treatment themselves, they are at the end of the funding power line and in reality have little or no say in the way services are delivered. This results in complete frustration at local level when their often strident and passionate voices are apparently ignored. For example, the official proposed fate of Omagh Hospital, which took the first call in the aftermath of the Omagh bombing, is contrary to extremely articulate and vociferous public wishes.

Case study

The Director of Clinical Services at Smalltown Infirmary agreed a waiting list initiative with key professionals. It included the following main points:

- Reduction in 'Did not attend' patients, by:
  - increasing recall intervals
  - reviewing need for recall and eliminating trivial reasons

- sending out appointment letters nearer the date of the appointment (previously three months' notice often led to patients forgetting)
- analysis of protocols used by outpatients staff to diminish patients' anxieties and to ensure that their examination and treatment were made as comfortable as possible.

- Reduction in waiting times for first appointments, by:

  - over summer months, considerably increased available resources on a once and for all basis
  - added clinical sessions at weekends and in the evenings to tackle backlog
  - streamlined clinic processes by increased levels of specialisation so that, where appropriate, patient through-put was increased
  - increased supplementary sessions, for example dietetics and physiotherapy, to improve overall patient welfare
  - added longer-term resources and clinics to maintain improvements.

- Reduction in waiting lists, by:
  The director could not influence those areas where there was a regional dependency on specialist care and treatment, but for treatments available on site, additional resources were committed to:

  - increase theatre availability in the evenings and at weekends
  - continue the extension of day surgery by using surgical ward space made vacant by increases in keyhole techniques
  - make further savings from a home care initiative for patients with acute chest problems, thus reducing admissions and possibly longer-term care and treatment.

3

Resource deficits

Shortages in the supply of money are not the sole cause of resource deficiencies. Certain key resources, for example highly qualified staff, can be scarce, particularly away from centres of excellence. Where there are shortages of key resources other than money, there will be an underspending in terms of budget but prolonged deficiencies will prejudice the viability of a service.

The issues

Budget managers cannot improve performance unless they identify the areas where there is a deficit in:

- the service provided
- the physical resources available
- the size of the budget that is allowed.

However, in the right circumstances, a service deficiency can be a means to attracting additional monies and this in turn may redress some of the physical resource problems, for example additional funding for key staff shortages (like doctors, dentists, social workers, nurses). This chapter gives a broad indication of:

- what to look for
- where to look for it
- what to do about it.

Introduction

In resource management it is imperative that managers are competent in managing consumption so that there is minimal waste in terms of both care and treatment, and in respect of the appropriate application of the means needed to carry out that care and treatment. It is a process that ranges from how we deal with patients, clients and the general public, through the utility of fixed resources such as buildings and equipment to the usage of people and materials.

The management, utility and mix of people, materials, equipment, estate, services, systems and structures provide the basis for efficiency and effectiveness. This constant challenge pervades the complete spectrum of management and operational activity and through it successful managers constantly make savings that in turn provide the flexibility to accomplish improvements.

This is a complex and time consuming process that consistently suggests − *appropriate action at the right time*. Below is a checklist of the main areas where these actions may be perceived.

Checklist of main resource management activity and interventions

▼ Developing a clear sense of mission through utilising the workplace as a management college and instilling core values in all members of staff.

▼ Reducing the insidious consequences of waste through constant vigilance and effort.

▼ Quickly identifying those assets that are nearing the end of their useful life.

▼ Noticing when resources are not being used effectively and taking appropriate remedial action to redistribute or otherwise improve resource utility.

▼ Identifying improvements and developments that will improve service quality.

▼ Finding an accurate cost for essential new or replacement items.

▼ Comprehending and making proper use of the systems that will facilitate replacement and/or new resources (planning, requisitioning and bidding).

▼ Developing savings programmes that properly reflect management activity.

This chapter deals mainly with those areas where there is a deficiency in the availability of resources or where there are detectable signals indicating that managers should take remedial action.

Resource profiles

General points of note are listed below.

- The spread of resources differs from trust to trust and from authority to authority.
- As a very broad generalisation, day-to-day running costs can be divided into two categories: staffing and other costs.
- Staffing accounts for between 70% and 80% of the total costs.
- In acute care, staffing costs will tend towards the 70% mark but this will depend on how much of the service has been contracted out. This has the effect of shifting costs out of direct payroll and into the category of goods and services.
- Other costs cover estate, drugs, Central/local Sterile Supply Departmental requirements (CSSD), equipment, furniture, heat, light, telephones, travel, laundry and a host of different types of materials and goods and services.

Broad examples of the day-to-day running costs for a variety of units are shown as pence in the pound in Tables 3.1–3.3.

Resource characteristics

In a climate of change a dynamic is present that requires flexibility in resource management whilst at the same time ensuring the stability of service

Table 3.1 The resources that the hospital pound buys

Resources	Pence
Staffing	
Medical	9
Nursing	36
Paramedics	5
Other	21
Other resources	
Estate	6
Goods and services	23
Total	100

Table 3.2   The resources that the community health service pound buys

Resources	Pence
Centres	16
Clinics	9
Visitors	17
Home nurses	38
Medical and dental schools	11
Laboratory services	9
Total	100

Table 3.3   The resources that the social services pound buys

Resources	Pence
Residential care	25
Day care	7
Learning difficulties	11
Fieldwork staff	17
Home helps	26
Other care	14
Total	100

provision. This is a delicate balance especially where there is fear that the future of a particular service, ward, department, residential home, hospital, etc. is in doubt. In these circumstances, there is always a danger that the resources supporting a service may become so mobile that people leave and replacements become harder and harder to find. This will impair service capacity and competence to a point where it may be judged hazardous to continue. Conversely, resources may be so stagnant that little or no change is possible (e.g. buildings lose their commercial value). In the cases of both mobility and stagnation, the scope for budgetary intervention is limited. There is therefore a need to balance flexibility against stability in resource structures.

Long resource life spans inevitably cause increasing running and maintenance costs. It is a phenomenon that, to a lesser extent, affects other resource categories like manpower, equipment, transport, etc. When these running costs exceed the cost of replacement, or are approaching it, the replacement option must be considered. This means that records of running

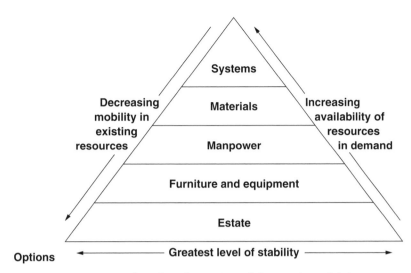

Figure 3.1   Resources (other than finance), mobility and availability structure.

costs must be maintained in such a way that they can be easily associated with the particular item so that a business case can be made. It is frequently necessary to compile this case from independent research. The main pressures on managers to keep the life span of a particular resource within manageable limits are a desire to have mobility and the cost of prolonging a life span beyond its realistic use. This is because of the need to identify and control resources adequately and implies that mechanisms must extend beyond the historical reporting system so that management intervention is not simply a reaction to cost trends but pervades every aspect of the management of the resources which are available.

The stability of an organisation's resource structure is illustrated in Figure 3.1, in which comparisons in the distribution of resource mobility between stable and flexible resource structures are graded according to potential life spans and availability (e.g. materials have a shorter life span than estate, but can usually be obtained more readily).

Tips from the front office

In stabilising existing services or where an alteration in the balance of care is required, the quality, consumption, availability and mobility of the resources used to support these services are key factors in creating and managing the movement needed to accommodate service change and improvement.

Sources of information on resource deficits

Built-in obsolescence, poor financial foresight, developments and discoveries, and long-term implications of deficiencies in management practice or appropriate usage may be the obvious causes of deficiencies in resources. But there are many other sources of information that managers should learn to utilise both in the context of creating an awareness of risk and in promoting a case for new or replacement items. These are often the result of inspection or audit and managers should be familiar with their content and concerns.

Below is a checklist of some of the areas where deficiencies in resource provision are highlighted.

Checklist of broad indicators of resource deficiency

▼   Regulatory or audit findings

— *Health, safety and other regulations.* Conformance with all regulations and advice to ensure the health and safety of patients, clients, staff and members of the general public are key requirements. Where any part of an operation has been found to be in any respect defective, managers will be taking steps to rectify the situation. However, where a major problem has been identified, for example evidence of extensive use of asbestos cladding, then the impact for service commissioning and provision in that area will be affected and that effect will have to be included in the business plan.

— *Audit.* The main sources of significant influence stem from the comptroller and auditor general whose reports to parliament may be the cause of select committee questions to the relevant officials. The results of these investigations are often the forerunner of amendments and adjustments to the way business is conducted. Value for money (VFM) scrutinies that cover a range of activities are examples of the type of topic under consideration. The results of some of these are quite well known. For examples, recruitment and advertising, residential accommodation, non-emergency ambulance service, central stores policy, the Supplies Service, Competitive Tendering Initiative. There may also be other more localised audit findings and criticism that require individual attention, for example application of charging regulations for private patients and road traffic accident patients.

— *Professional inspection.* Accreditation for training and other professional requirements are subject to the inspection and assessment by a variety of professional bodies. In the course of this process, deficiencies in patient or client care are often detected, for example beds placed in areas not designated for care or treatment (corridors are the cause of frequent complaint). These throw up important quality considerations which, if prevalent, will again have to be taken into account in the business plan.

▼ *Ombudsman and other commissioners.* Managers will be concerned at the levels of criticism of their record in the execution of statutory and other regulatory obligations as far as recruitment and management of both staff and patients/clients are concerned. Managers need to follow up any complaints and ensure that the correct approach is adopted in every case so that unfortunate incidents are kept to an absolute minimum. They will want to take steps to eliminate any loopholes that may exist in their employment policy and administration. In all cases managers must make maximum use of conciliatory and mediatory facilities.

▼ *Liability considerations.* As well as being a cost to the organisation, unsettled compensation claims or legal liabilities are indicators of the level of negligence. Beyond the normal control and disciplinary mechanisms lie the circumstances in which the incidents occurred. Managers need to be acutely aware of these underlying factors and to take steps to see that proper risk assessment and quality control and management procedures are implemented in the future.

▼ *External pressure groups.* These can include a number of vested interests that may or may not find expression through the operation of the local health councils. They often represent important public concerns and must never be ignored. Often the efforts of groups worried about perceived deficiencies in service provision find tangible expression in significant fund raising. This is an area in which relevant managers need to take an interest. As well as being useful future allies, voluntary group efforts can be complementary to funding deficits.

Asset review

Managers need to balance the information gleaned from the above list with a constant factual review of deficiencies in the resources they have or need.

This must cover all resources, including staffing, and should take account of the expected working life of each individual category as described in the next section.

Identifying deficient physical resources

The expected working life of all resources, including staffing levels and competence, in the context of their localised environment should be identified and tested against maintenance costs and a timetable of replacement needs. The life span of items, goods, services and materials can be fairly accurately assessed and, although usually having long-term implications, staffing too has obvious and known working life implications.

In the case of staffing, it is also possible to identify other indicators that can clearly show low morale which is having a detrimental effect on overall performance. This is dealt with in more detail in the relevant section below.

The life span inventory can then be reviewed further in the light of current developments, repairs, sickness, etc. to see whether obsolescence is a threat that goes beyond the particular and pervades or infects the future of the whole unit.

Staffing

It is well known that health and social care provision is extremely labour intensive. Around 70% of running costs are devoted to staffing and managers must ensure that working conditions and expectations are at reasonable standards and levels. One of the essential aspects of this is ensuring that staff on the payroll are available for work.

From earliest times, morale has been generally recognised as one of the key factors that facilitate or diminish an organisation's capacity to be successful. It is important to keep an efficient team together and to avoid those pressures and rumours that cause dissatisfaction.

The ability to recognise and improve poor or low morale is therefore a crucial management attribute and taking proper measures will enhance performance. In addition, managers must bear in mind the developing nature of essential health and social staff skills: thus they need to develop a programme that embraces those new skills through training and other additions. This all comes at a cost.

Below is a checklist of key indicators of a lowering of morale.

Checklist of key indicators of a lowering of morale

▼ *Staff turnover.* Few organisations or units have a full complement of staff. Turnover is part of the normal expectation of staff management and the rates will vary according to the type of organisation. However, high rates of staff turnover coupled with difficulties in recruitment are indicators of a lowering of morale and managers must take appropriate steps to correct this trend.

▼ *Likely future vacancies.* A review of benefits and deficiencies in key areas, together with imminent retirements, needs to be carried out. This exercise will show the degree of resource mobility and will be a determining factor as far as timescales are concerned. It is also essential at this stage to review any obligatory safeguards and other confidence-building measures for the purposes of assuring staff and public in their separate consultative processes.

▼ *Sickness and absenteeism levels.* Health and social care organisations have well-developed systems that follow up staff with long-term or frequent health problems. However, the reason for high incidences of sickness or absenteeism may lie beneath the surface and may reflect a general unease with working conditions, persistent negative rumours and poor management techniques and reputation.

▼ *Workloads and dependencies.* Where workloads and dependencies are increasing there are limits to the amount of extra work staff can reasonably absorb. The point at which toleration diminishes will depend very much on the spirit of the department, but clearly long hours with no respite against a background of escalating expectations are potentially hazardous for everyone concerned. Managers must take these matters seriously.

▼ *Complaints.* Again, a certain level of complaint is normal. But where there is an increasing number from patients/clients, or from internal sources including staff, they must be thoroughly investigated and resolved. In order to establish base lines and later comparisons, records should be kept of the number, type and source of complaints.

▼ *Claims for negligence.* Detailed records are already available for these incidents and the subsequent action taken. Managers should be familiar with their impact as far as increases or decreases are concerned.

Tips from the front office

Managers must be sure that any action they are going to take is compatible with an overall strategy. For example, the application of an over zealous policy on sickness may be counterproductive where turbulence in the workforce already exists — first tackle the reasons for turbulence.

An increasing stock of vacancies may actually be of assistance where a part of the organisation is to be restructured.

Below is a checklist of steps aimed at creating conditions for improved morale.

Checklist of steps to improve morale

▼ *Establish performance database* for sickness, absenteeism, accidents, complaints, negligence, mistakes, fraud, deliberate vandalism, etc. and any other untoward events. Obtain comparisons from similar departments and/or other organisations. Keep records of disciplinary matters. Assess the state of morale based on reliable data.

▼ *Pay.* Make sure that salaries and wages payable to staff are correct and up to date. Constantly inaccurate pay due to the receipt of late documentation can be debilitating.

   – Maintain the flow of necessary documentation for all stages in employment, inception, overtime, special duty payments, etc. Late or irregular submission will affect your budget statement, which will not be accurate either.
   – Remember that computerisation reduces drudgery but does not replace intelligence, so make sure that your submissions are accurate.
   – Be aware of system security weaknesses and check names against facts.
   – Improve communication by networking with other key departmental heads, personnel, etc.

▼ *Competence and rewards.* Ensure that staff are properly rewarded. Meanness is not a money saver in the longer term.

   – Standardise and rate methodologies appropriate to each task.
   – Develop specialist skill levels and integrate with appropriate responsibilities, etc.

- Commensurately reward staff according to workload demands and do not allow staff to consistently work unreasonable hours.
- Do not confuse excessive speed of task completion with efficiency and effectiveness.
- Prepare succession plans.

▼ *Team building creates staff awareness.* Teams are not created through the employment process. You have to work at it.

- Become involved in the recruitment and induction of your own staff.
- Ensure that your training programme is appropriate to each level of skill.
- Get involved in the induction processes of other disciplines.
- Know your own staff on a personal basis.
- Divide and apportion workloads to specialist teams.
- Structure teams to reflect defined responsibilities.

▼ *Training.* Induction and ongoing training programmes are important assets in the drive to improve morale. Make sure that feelings and complaints expressed in the classroom are properly channelled into the system so their impact can be assessed.

- Utilise the workplace as a management college for teams and individuals.
- Foster core values and instil a sense of mission.

▼ *Communication and assurance.* An open system of communications and information will help dispel any adverse rumours or at worst will facilitate the management of bad news.

▼ *Set and/or agree clear and achievable objectives.* Conflicting or, taking account of resource levels, impossible objectives diminish morale. Ensure a sense of direction, give and get commitment — agreed mission statements are often efficacious.

▼ *Discipline.* Make sure the organisation's code of conduct is reasonable, appropriate and acceptable and that it is applied impartially.

- Promote and accept only the highest standards of behaviour.
- Develop and foster an atmosphere of mutual respect.
- Ensure that maximum privacy and confidentiality are accorded to all.
- Deal with all complaints and criticisms pesonally. Be quietly persistent.
- Take steps to correct deficiency and keep progress under review.

▼ *Process quality*. Foster a culture of doing the *right* thing *first* time, *every* time.

▼ *Pride in the deparment or organisation*. Generate pride in a good reputation through team working and the provision of team figures for key performance indicators. Encourage ideas for general improvement and for developments that will lead to expansion of the customer base.

▼ *Equality*. Ensure that all employees, from the bottom to the top, are treated with equal respect and are paid according to the work they do, not who or what they are.

▼ *Conditions of employment*. As well as rewards and remuneration, conditions can be systematically improved by enhancing the working environment so that it is appropriate to the tasks undertaken. Health and safety, cleanliness, lighting, heat, decoration, state of repair, and canteen and toilet facilities are simple considerations that affect workforce morale.

▼ *Awkward customer relations*. High customer/client expectation, coupled with the frustration of dealing with a large and apparently impersonal organisation, has in recent years produced the customer rage phenomenon. Staff who have to deal with such difficulties may suffer a loss of morale and management must take a proactive role in providing support.

Tips from the front office

A plan based on a survey of the above factors and converted into acceptability criteria can readily be drawn up but its implementation needs to be measured against both the databases and observations so that genuine increase in morale is seen to be matched by improvements in performance.

As a morale-boosting measure and as a sustained effort to improve and develop competences and communication skills of the individual, the use of the workplace as a management college has proved to be a cost-effective option. Improvements in practice depend on attention being clearly focused on the individual and his context. This means concentrating on the needs of the *individual*, the *organisation* and the *individual in the organisation*. This is a low-cost, high-performance option that can easily be applied to staff development in the workplace. Below is a checklist of pick-and-mix attributes.

Checklist of attributes and benefits of the workplace as a management college

▼ *Integrated in-house management development*

- a variety of models that benefit the individual, the organisation and the individual in the organisation without compromising any aspect
- provides scope for growth from within
- provides in-house opportunities for small to large numbers of staff from a wide range of disciplines or conversely it can be both selective and exclusive
- can easily embrace a wide range of initiatives from action learning sets, support for individual projects, quality issues and the more formal classroom style of delivery

▼ *Flexibility*

- workplace environment as the main focus for valuation and improvement
- to determine individual developmental speeds and complexities
- relative importance attributed to individual goals and ambitions.

▼ *Management commitment.* A tripartite continuum that embraces the manager, the individual and appropriate external providers is an essential component.

▼ *Academic partnership.* Although the essential task is the development of individuals in their job, it must also cover professional and academic requirements.

▼ *Accreditation and quality assurance*

- an accreditation of mutually agreed levels of attainment
- internal certification and recognition are key morale boosters
- acceptability criteria that can be identified and used to enhance performance.

▼ *Review and amendment process.* The involvement of potential course participants in the planning, implementation and audit of the initiative is a crucial element.

Tips from the front office

▼   The promotion of excellence in management practice through continuous review and modification in the light of experience is an attractive proposition.

▼   Overstimulation of high-flying potential can create frustration, dissatisfaction and instability in the workplace.

▼   There is always a danger that overemphasis on academia can prejudice practitioner culture.

▼   Incremental remuneration and conditions commensurate with improvements.

Estate

With the value of the health and social care estate estimated at around £40 billion, capital spending on new units, etc. around £2 billion annually and the cost of day-to-day maintenance of most units running at about 6% of the total revenue budget, it makes sense to ensure that these assets that we all take for granted are fully utilised and not subject to unnecessary abuse.

In addition to a review of the quantity, utility and condition of the grounds and buildings, other estate services such as heat, power and light (2% of day-to-day running costs) and telephones (1%) etc. should also be included.

Estate managers will have overall responsibility for the maintenance and improvement of the estate, including grounds, and they execute their complex tasks in a variety of ways. However, even where funds are available there is a considerable degree of formality to the execution of new proposals and service managers have to bear this in mind.

For anything other than routine maintenance where the response time should be reasonable, proposed new works need to be scheduled into a programme of priorities. This suggests that service managers must recognise the likely delays that will be involved in fulfilling their proposals, if indeed their proposals are accepted. This has an important bearing on the feasibility of new ideas and it can be frustrating if managers do not take these limitations into their initial calculations. Below is a checklist of main headings.

**Checklist of main estate management categories of work
(waiting time for work to be completed is inferred from
the relative complexity)**

▼ *Day-to-day maintenance.* This can take various forms ranging from
  direct responses to requests for repairs, through to a programme of
  planned preventative maintenance which involves regular checks on
  lights, plumbing, locks, etc. by qualified tradespeople. To cope with
  this workload, estate mangers

  – usually have at their disposal directly employed labour and
    directly purchased materials
  – may also have sums of money in reserve to deal with backlogs of
    maintenance and for small once-and-for-all projects, like a paint-
    ing programme that could be subcontracted out at appropriate
    and convenient times.

▼ *Larger-scale works programmes.* This would be for schemes of more
  complex work that may extend over longer periods and which
  require substantial funding, for example extensive replacement of
  roofs or major electrical rewiring schemes. As such work could not
  be undertaken by existing staff, it would have to be arranged
  through a formal tendering and contracting process and adminis-
  tered through project management techniques which should almost
  certainly involve the departmental or unit head.

▼ *Major capital works projects.* This is usually the heading under which
  new building is included. It involves big money and long timescales,
  and, because of the technical, legal and project management
  commitments is managed externally by the health authority. If the
  proposal is for a new hospital for example, then inevitably years
  will pass from the initial idea to completion. It may be that due to
  shortage of capital funds, the eventual selected provider will be
  determined through the Public Finance Initiative. This means that
  when the project is finally handed over for use, responsibility for
  future maintenance will usually lie with the private provider.

Tips from the front office

Individual managers must ensure that the premises they occupy are
being used effectively and not abused. This means that in order to be

sure that their domain is up to date or at least within the programme of works, individual managers have to keep in contact with the estates division to check on progress.

The checklist below provides guidance on the places to look for deficiencies or improvements.

Checklist of estate deficiency considerations

▼ *Utility*

  – Check that the use of space is appropriate to need, i.e. that offices, stores, toilets and bathrooms, treatment rooms, public areas and other patient/client areas are occupied as intended.
  – Where there is an over- or underutilisation of all or any space in a particular category, this may be a benefit or a deficiency depending on plans.
  – If there is to be a development or a redecoration or refurbishment programme, for example, then vacant space can be a benefit.
  – Where workloads have fallen and certain spaces are no longer needed then steps must be taken to reallocate.
  – Where there is overcrowding, additional space is required.
  – In resource terms, deficiencies occur in both cases. Redistribution, re-designation and possibly additional works to make areas suitable for different client or patient groups may be necessary.

▼ *Transport links*. Check out transport links to make sure that they are appropriate to the current or intended use of the estate and consider what proposals are necessary to make improvements.
▼ *Car parking/grounds*. Check that they are suitable for the current or proposed use. This includes gardens, car parking, rest areas and other outdoor amenities.
▼ *Services*. Check to make sure that services such as water, heat, power, light, telephones and specific clinical or other requirements can be and are being consistently met.
▼ *Condition*. The actual condition of the estate is the aspect with which most managers become obsessed if the need for urgent repairs is essential.

- The most obvious – weatherproofing, breakages, plumbing and electrical failures – should all receive priority treatment.
- Some repairs will receive attention only in response to constant pressure from the departmental manager.
- After a time, whether or not there are plenty of plausible excuses, no action may result in invisibility, for example a long line of cracked floor tiles in outpatients probably indicates that the concrete subfloor is faulty and that eliminates simple remedial work.
- At some point towards the end of a building's useful life, a decision has to be taken about its future.

▼ *Hazards*. Because issues of health and safety receive such high priority from authorities and trusts, this paragraph is to be taken as an indicator only. However, in a manager's busy day risks from fire, noxious substances, food distribution and poor practices can easily be overlooked and may even be inadvertently condoned. For example, as an energy conservation measure reduced lighting levels in stairwells can be hazardous from the accident point of view as well as posing a potential security risk.

▼ *Fire precautions* must have priority over resource management considerations. Managers must be scrupulous about compliance with all regulations and be attentive to practices that potentially block doorways or keep them shut or open. They must also take care to be up to date and vigilant about possible evacuation routes, particularly where dependency is on the increase.

▼ *Impact of planned works*. Managers must be constantly alert to the impact that proposed works schemes will have on their service provision. They must also be careful to follow up imminent stage deadlines on their own proposals especially at the start and finish.

Materials, furniture and equipment

This is a complex category that covers all resources that cannot be categorised as either staff or estate. Mostly materials, especially drugs, are for almost immediate consumption and the supply lines have to reflect this urgency. On the other hand furniture and equipment will not be immediately available. Indeed considerable delays may be experienced in obtaining furniture and equipment. These delays are due to a number of factors, noted in the checklist below.

Checklist of delay factors in obtaining furniture and equipment

▼   Shortage of funds means that demands should be met on a priority basis.
▼   Approval of proposals that arise from the introduction of a potentially new service can be time consuming.
▼   Complex rules governing large-scale equipment like x-ray machinery can mean a prolonged process of option appraisal.
▼   Once a request is in the system, larger purchases are subject to tendering and contracting procedures.
▼   Suppliers may experience delays in meeting demand.
▼   The time allowed may expire.

Tips from the front office

▼   Make a plan for the assessment of the condition and replacement for all furniture and equipment.
▼   Allow lifespans of three years for electrical equipment and ten years for furniture and furnishings.
▼   Ensure that servicing occurs at stipulated intervals.
▼   Check out down times and the mounting cost of repairs.
▼   Keep up to date with new developments and the changing availability of money.
▼   Will your proposal save time and money? Be specific about this.
▼   Start early with your development list.

The fact that managers are almost unaware of problems in obtaining consumables is a tribute to the effective way in which this works. Materials flow in many directions throughout an organisation. It is crucial that supply and distribution processes to secure the right quantity and quality at the right price are maintained without the need to stockpile. Unfortunately, regardless of the size and scope of the operation, active participation in these arrangements and the release of appropriate regulatory documentation are not seen as priorities by departmental managers. Below is a checklist of essential activities and tips, which will have an effect on budgetary performance.

Checklist of tips for regulating and managing materials handling

Do

▼ Participate in all materials user forums (MUFs) aimed at standardising specifications and obtaining value for money (VFM).

▼ Encourage creativity in supply chain management and note any complaints from operatives.

▼ Facilitate new product trials and comment positively. Engage properly with product evaluation teams (PETs).

▼ Contribute to the pre- and post-contract negotiating process.

▼ Generate order communications in accordance with agreed time-scales and methodologies.

▼ Check all goods received immediately for quality and quantity.

▼ Immediately notify any doubts about contractor compliance.

▼ Clear all queries and documentation without delay.

▼ Contribute fully to review processes.

Don't

▼ Waste energy and time on hostility to supply chain initiatives with unattractive objectives.

▼ Economise at the expense of health and safety.

▼ Ignore complaints or warnings about potential hazards.

▼ Take unnecessary risks.

▼ Stockpile. Keep stocks to a minimum. Overstocking provides temptation to pilfer and is costly to maintain.

▼ Allow materials to become out of date.

Tips from the front office

▼ Quality is compliance with the appropriate specification – it is *not* usually the most expensive item.

▼ Quantities should always be exact: make sure you are using the correct units i.e. one only, tens, dozens, hundreds, gross, etc.

▼ Check out the efficacy of just-in-time (JIT) stock management systems.

▼ Where stocks are maintained at low levels, timely deliveries are essential.

Prioritising and bidding for resources

When confronted with competing demands for larger-scale replacements or for new developments, managers have to have a rational system for determining the order or scale of need that each proposal attracts. This matter has been previously discussed in some detail in *Managing Health and Social Care: essential checklists for frontline staff*.[1] However, below is a checklist of key guidance points.

Checklist of resource priority guidelines

You can prioritise demands according to the following rough criteria by giving a notional score. This will allow you to see which are likely to succeed. (*See* Chapter 6 for more details on rating intangible benefits.)

▼ *Financial planning cycle*. Where large amounts of money are involved make sure your bid is submitted so that it conforms with the financial planning cycle.

▼ *Strategic direction*. Ensure that your projects are in harmony with the overall direction that your organisation has chosen (see the checklist below).

▼ *Additional funding*. Look out for extra monies becoming available for cherished initiatives.

▼ *Health and safety issues*. These are always of serious concern and bids or demands that improve conditions can attract a better rating.

▼ *Cost*. Depending upon the scale of the cost and other competition for scarce funds, this can have a detrimental effect on success. Think of breaking up the bid into workable component parts or see whether other options instead of a straight purchase are available. (*See* Chapter 6.)

▼ *Delivery*. Can your proposals be delivered within a reasonable timescale? A long lead time or potential delays can be mean unacceptability.

Checklist of strategic directions for health and social care

In addition to the general trends towards a continued alteration in the balance of health and social care in favour of more appropriate levels and modes of delivery, and the development of partnerships between health and social services to improve the continuity of care, etc. improvement in overall core services in the following categories will continue to be encouraged:

▼   maternal and child health
▼   accidents and trauma
▼   mental health
▼   circulatory diseases
▼   cancers
▼   respiratory diseases
▼   physical and sensory disability
▼   rehabilitation to higher degrees of independence
▼   child and family care, especially in the movement of children out of residential or fostering care and into a more stable family situation such as offered by adoption
▼   community care.

Key action points

▼   In a climate of constant change, never be surprised at any deficit you discover.
▼   Discover deficits before it is too late to take the proper action.
▼   Be prepared for all eventualities.
▼   Be systematically vigilant of the condition of your internal and external environment.
▼   Prioritise your demands and make sure they conform with current philosophy and development.
▼   Make your bid at the correct time.

Reference

1   Bryans W (2004) *Managing Health and Social Care: essential checklists for frontline staff.* Radcliffe Medical Press, Oxford.

4

Quality, expectation and costs

The complex means whereby the ever-increasing demand for a wide range of clinical options and different methodologies for the provision of social care is balanced with the reality of scarce resources is based on basic economic principles. This balance is reflected in the strenuous efforts that are made to ensure equity (not always successfully) and effectiveness. Supply, demand, competition, cost and price have all been introduced to the health and social care vocabulary. This chapter gives an overview of how these principles are applied and provides guidance on how managers might respond.

The issues

- One of the continual refinements in the way money is made available is the recent announcement of the introduction of national tariffs for the NHS – just when it was thought that the internal market had disappeared.
- Comprehending how this has come about and the likely consequences will help reduce the dissonance so frequently experienced when either allocating or analysing the distribution of wealth throughout the spectrum of health and social care.
- This chapter concentrates on the criteria and measurements that can be applied to improve quality and performance. It includes:

  – an outline of the theory of supply and demand
  – how cost is defined, with examples
  – factors that affect cost and ways that costs may be reduced.

Introduction

Whilst the range and scope of treatment options spiral upwards and the general demand upon health and social care increases, it becomes ever easier to criticise both simple day-to-day resource management and investment decisions. Similarly, the methods that are used to calculate the amount paid to a provider have always been under close scrutiny. Consequences of decisions or systems, including those that might at the time have appeared trivial, can develop into sources of bitter acrimony.

Over the past couple of decades the gradual introduction of simple economic concepts such as price, cost and volume indicates a greater reliance on the practical benefits to be derived from a rational approach to these complex problems.

One important, though not exclusive, problem relates to the application of historical and often unverified data to the here-and-now. Doubtless the inflexibility of the NHS finance regime, together with the financial year time limit approach to budgets and spending, diminish managers' strategic capacity and tend to create a culture of short-termism.

There may also be conflict of and confusion about purpose on the part of both managers and clinicians. Such factors are not necessarily commensurate with a rational approach to decision-making. Indeed, such uncertainty and ambiguity sometimes typify much of a complex organisation's function and tend to diminish effective decision-making in the context of a rational model.

It is therefore a natural response to hedge the allocation and decision-making processes with sometimes piecemeal safeguards. Because of the usual time constraints on spending these can and often do result in administrative stagnation and the loss of an opportunity. The recent introduction of payment for particular procedures based on a national tariff will cause anxiety for those whose costs exceed the amount paid.

It will be no surprise that the application of these so called 'rational' solutions to resource allocation dilemmas at local level is going to be difficult. This chapter provides accessible and useful guidance to the understanding and application of the principles as efficacious influences on commissioners and providers at every link in the resource chain.

Supply and demand

The connection between quality and cost is well established in the public consciousness – 'You get what you pay for ...' and more pessimistically, 'You get *only* what you pay for ...' These are sentiments that pervade the modern shopper's psyche. They contain the semipermanent truths that govern availability. Even in wartime and in the immediate postwar era, with the harsh realities of scarcity reflected in rationing, money may have assisted the procurement of desirable items on the black market.

Thus, in prevailing circumstances, the highest bidder may be able to coax the supplier into providing an item or service that may be scarce. However, availability is as much about internal as external factors. A provider may be restricted by the cost of internal optimum capacity – cost is directly related to volume.

Supply

As volume increases, the supply cost increases but the rate of increase slows until optimum capacity is reached. At lower volumes the rate of increasing costs is higher because the provider has to carry the additional burden of spare capacity. This phenomenon will be dealt with in more detail as the chapter progresses. A simplified case where quality is maintained at a certain level is shown in Figure 4.1.

Demand

Abundance in the years following the austerity of wartime has fostered and encouraged the desire for all the material benefits that money can buy. Although, amongst other factors, a market may become saturated or tastes change, part of the generation of demand can be attributed to a reduction in cost to purchasers. Thus, in simplified terms and within limits, as costs fall demand increases. This is illustrated in Figure 4.2.

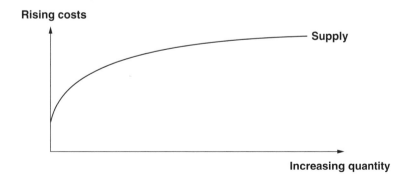

Figure 4.1   Supply and cost.

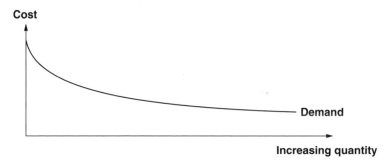

Figure 4.2   Demand and cost.

At zero cost or a tendency towards zero, a saturation demand may be created that may never ultimately be met.

The classic theory

The respective levels of supply and demand depend on and vary with cost. Cost depends on and varies with movements in supply and demand. In any set of variable circumstances, but at constant quality, it is therefore possible to predict where all the conditions are satisfied. This is illustrated in Figure 4.3 below.

   Where there is a significant demand beyond the point at which the price has settled, a gap develops between the ability to supply and demand. This

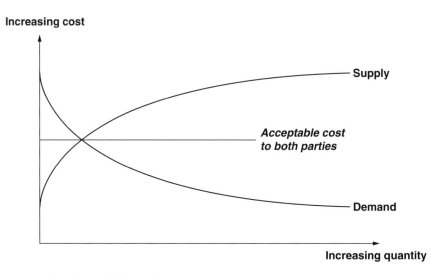

Figure 4.3   Supply and demand curves.

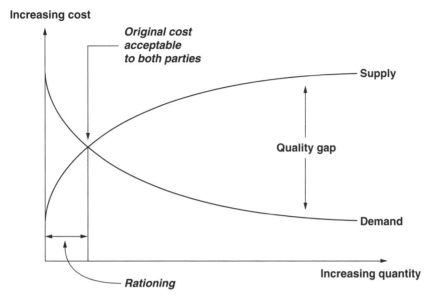

Figure 4.4   Supply and demand gap.

regulation and potential for the rationing of volume obviously affect the perception of quality, as illustrated in Figure 4.4.

Tips from the front office

▼   Quality in terms of volume can often be obtained at an agreed cost.
▼   Limited volume can mask underutilised resources.
▼   Low volumes can be a threat to safety due to lack of practice.
▼   High volumes may also be unsafe because of overwork.
▼   Scarcity and rationing can be symptomatic of a shortage of cash.
▼   Each factor in the equation is inextricably linked to the others.

Practical aspects of cost and workload

The famous example of men digging a trench illustrates the various factors that influence cost. Depending on the size of the trench and other factors, increasing the number of men and/or other resources will improve matters. In simple arithmetic, two men could do the job twice as fast as one and three could complete it three times as fast as one.

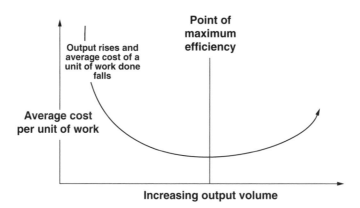

Figure 4.5 Simplified average cost curve.

However, this ignores the impact of specialisation, team work and efficiency. For example, in the case of three men, one might be responsible for digging, one for shovelling and one for barrowing and wheeling away. In theory, the job would be completed much more quickly. In other words, the rate at which the units of work were completed would increase and, although the total amount spent would also increase, the cost per unit would fall.

As more men are added, efficiency would continue to increase up to a maximum. At this point, the site would become so cluttered that output would suffer. *See* Figure 4.5.

Total cost increases according to work done but the average cost falls until a point of maximum efficiency is reached when the average cost would begin to rise.

As well as the availability of labour in the correct proportions, there may be other constraints on output volume or work done. There may not be enough work or due to other circumstances the work may become unnecessary. On the other hand, some unexpected difficulty may occur that leads to a reassessment of the position.

These factors become critical when output falls on either side of the point of maximum efficiency and then, from a financial point of view, the management system is at a disadvantage. What can be done?

In the case of a work shortage, instead of paying off workers the manager might try to take on other work or amalgamate with someone else who requires extra resources.

Where there is too much work or where it has become too difficult, then the decision might be taken to hire or purchase mechanical help, thus reducing labour costs to one operator and one driver.

Provided there are accurate and reliable data, these criteria can be applied to health and social care. However, in order to be effective managers need to be competent in verification, analysis, interpretation and intervention. The checklist below summarises what they need to know.

Checklist of management cost competences

Check:

▼   what the data mean and whether they are verifiable
▼   whether the data can be enhanced or developed to suit specialist needs
▼   what corrections need to be incorporated to improve the data
▼   how to determine whether the department/unit is efficient in financial terms
▼   how to improve output or increase the resources available
▼   when to change the way of working to reflect current developments
▼   when and how to obtain additional investment in modern equipment.

Cost, workload and budget

Where the acceptable cost at a defined level of dependency for a particular number of patients or clients treated is agreed, the budget allocated for that set of circumstances can be easily calculated. These relationships are illustrated in Figure 4.6.

The budget can be calculated according to the specification for a range of workload values. As workload increases, the average cost per unit will fall until a point of optimum efficiency is reached. At any particular point, the total cost or the value of the budget is found by multiplying the workload (w) by the average agreed cost (c) for that dependency level.

Sometimes managers are inclined to ignore this relationship and seek savings from existing arrangements. Where a specification is part of a contract, this must be changed in order to comply with revised funding. This does not mean that managers should cease their pursuit of more cost-effective ways of working. Also, where otiose resources are perceived particularly in connection with estate, it does not follow that with a commensurate increase

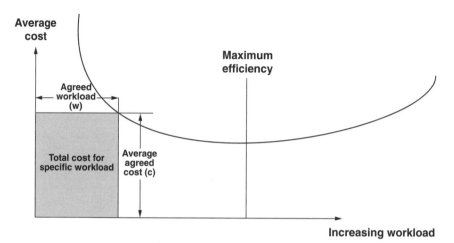

Figure 4.6 Average cost and workload.

in staffing these can be brought into use safely without the dangers of a knock-on effect further along the dependency chain or of hazards remaining undetected in the creation of unsafe practices. Below is a checklist of Do's and Don'ts.

Checklist of guidelines

▼ Don't be tempted to ignore these relationships and seek savings from existing arrangements.

▼ Where a specification is part of a contract, this must be changed in order to comply with revised funding.

▼ Never cease the pursuit of more cost-effective ways of working.

▼ Don't pressurise staff or use other resources so that they fall into a persistent cycle of overwork: they will burnout, make mistakes and become less focused.

▼ Identify resources that are not in full use, then put them to work or decommission them.

▼ Look out for improvements or developments that will be more cost effective.

▼ Don't introduce or tolerate unsafe practices or other hazards.

▼ Where resources are perceived to be not in full use, particularly in connection with estate, it does not follow that with a commensurate increase in staffing these can be brought into use safely without the dangers of a knock-on effect further along the dependency chain or of hazards remaining undetected in the creation of unsafe practices.

Case studies

- In St Bedifuls some operating theatres are not used during the evenings, at night and at weekends. Taking account of cleansing and other maintenance requirements, more of these could be brought into use with the introduction of shift systems. However, this would introduce accommodation and other problems elsewhere where spare capacity was not so obvious, e.g. wards, etc.
- Many community resource centres and sheltered workshops in Bigtown close during unsociable hours. These could be used for increases in the volume of respite care provision so that there is better use of spare capacity.

Comparative costs

Comparative costs are used to compare the financial performance of one unit with another. Table 4.1 below shows what they look like.

Table 4.1 Example of comparative costs (in thousands of pounds)

	Facilities						
	A	B	C	D	E	F	Total
Overall costs							
Payroll	7	19	32	39	45	66	208
Other expenditure	3	8	13	17	25	30	96
Total cost	10	27	45	56	70	96	304
Work units	1	3	5	7	10	12	38
Average cost per unit							
Payroll	7	6.3	6.4	5.6	4.5	5.5	5.5
Other expenditure	3	2.7	2.6	2.4	2.4	2.5	2.5
Total average cost	10	9	9	8	6.9	8	8

In the past, where a unit has been near the bottom of the league table, such comparisons have tended to stimulate improvements. In future, because of the introduction of national tariffs, poor results will need radical action to achieve better performance. From Table 4.1 it can be seen that overall:

- facility A is the smallest in terms of productivity and the most financially inefficient
- F is the largest facility but not the most financially efficient
- the lowest average cost per unit of work is achieved by facility E at £6.9
- the highest average cost per unit of work is attributed to the smallest unit, A, at £10
- if A was closed and the work transferred to E, presuming the same average cost could be sustained, the savings would only be £3,000 (10 minus 7, multiplied by 1000) – unless they were close together, probably not worth the hassle!
- facility C may be more vulnerable with a potential saving of £10,000
- if this example was the cost of a very minor procedure and the national tariff was £7 per case, then the loss for A and C would be similar.

On closer examination, facility E's payroll costs are markedly lower at £4.5 than the average (£5.5), whilst the cost of other expenses is the same. This would suggest that either E has found a radical new way of dealing with cases that saves considerable time or there has been a mistake in attributing payroll costs to the procedure.

This raises the question of how payroll costs are arrived at. It is possible to identify the statistics relating to particular cases with relative ease but no member of staff signs in and out when they change from one procedure to another. So what methodology has been used? Is it based upon a sample or an estimate? This is an area that needs further investigation. Remember that if an estimate or other type of apportionment is found to be inaccurate, a reworking of the attributed cost will have an effect on some other aspect of service.

Alteration in the balance and the budget

When they have time to reflect, managers are often surprised at the dramatic way in which health and social care has changed and been changed over the years. The truth of the matter is that when a clinical or care breakthrough occurs dependency in that particular sphere tends to decrease or often disappears and the need for dedicated resources evaporates without prior approval or management.

Checklist of examples

▼   Elimination of the need for hospitals solely dedicated to the care and treatment of those suffering from tuberculosis.

▼   Introduction and development of transplant techniques.
▼   Polio and other forms of immunisation.
▼   Continued advances in preventative medicine.
▼   Advances in the treatment of cancer and its management.
▼   Improvement in drug therapy for people suffering from various
     forms of mental illness and the gradual movement away from long-
     stay institutional care.
▼   Developments in the treatment of infertility and advances in
     conception techniques.
▼   Reductions in hospital stays through advances in a variety of
     techniques such as keyhole and day surgery.

All these examples, which indicate a different and improved direction, have
financial consequences which must be reflected in the amount of resources
dedicated at each level and on the budget that is available.

Looking back at Figure 4.6, the budget should be the agreed total cost for
the agreed amount of work to be undertaken at an agreed standard. However,
managers must be constantly aware that the balance of care is continually
shifting in favour of a more appropriate form of care. This means shorter stays
at any stage but a concentration on higher dependency levels. It also means
that community care will have greater numbers at higher dependency levels.

In Figure 4.7 the 'old budget' for dependency level (i) has to be recalculated
to reflect the requirements of dependency level (ii).

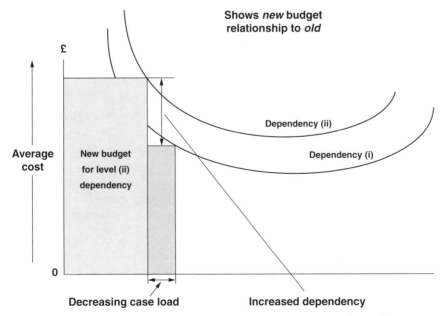

Figure 4.7   Alteration in the balance of care and increasing dependency.

It can be seen that a reduction in workload with a greater degree of dependency has resulted in a shift of costs away from the optimum position. In order to survive in these circumstances, the budget manager would have to obtain a greater market share and/or rationalise beds or places, etc. or have the budget recalculated to arrive at the correct amount.

Where case mixes are more complex than this situation, a separate budget calculation would be necessary for each one – if the detail could be identified. There would, nevertheless, have to be a number of assumptions relating to the apportionment of fixed and other costs. This process becomes more and more difficult as the system is refined and there is a danger that sight may be lost of the main objectives. This aspect is a major problem for providers who wish to move away from volume costs and towards a more sophisticated procedure-based contractual arrangement.

The main connections between workload, dependency and cost are listed in the checklist below.

Checklist of terminology that links dependency, workload and cost

▼ *Dependency*, as an aspect of quality, must be managed through an infrastructure designed to both stimulate improvement and maintain standards. In many respects measurements are reflections on intangible benefits:

   – the system must be cost effective
   – intangible benefits must be weighted to reflect equity
   – the whole range of measurement issues must be considered
   – basic facts are contained in readily available statistical tables.

▼ *Total cost* or resource consumption is closely linked to the workload or volume of patients or clients treated or cared for. It is a mixture of two elements – the *fixed cost* and the *variable cost*. In perfect conditions (where there is no ageing, obsolescence or sudden changes in care and treatment regimes) a number of phenomena occur:

   – *Fixed costs* are usually thought of as the costs incurred in purchasing and/or maintaining estate and equipment. In the case of care and treatment, sometimes absolute minimum levels of staff and materials are also included. This cost will remain the same until maximum capacity is reached. After that, additional estate and equipment will be needed.
   – *Variable costs*, which are those costs directly influenced by the volume of work undertaken, gradually increase with increases

of workload. These are usually thought of as including payroll and materials.

▼ *Workload* varies with dependency and it is important therefore to compare like with like.
▼ *Average cost* is usually expressed as an average cost per item, i.e. the total cost divided by the total quantity within the same workload category.
▼ *Cost mobility*. Costs are said to have cost mobility in two directions. First there is the mobility already described, where there is movement because of increases in volume. The other type occurs during the time-scale in which the cost is incurred. Thus mobility can be influenced either by the passage of time or by the volume handled. These two factors have important consequences when we begin to examine how costs can best be controlled.
▼ *Predictability*. Although it might be reasonably expected that those costs which are described as fixed do not display any variation characteristics, in fact, for a number of reasons they are subject to fluctuation. In other words, despite the fact that the total cost is constant, either the supply of the fixed cost items may be irregular or the demand for payment may not be made in equal increments.

Matching care to cost

There have been many arguments favouring the reshaping of health and social care to help older and vulnerable people to regain their independence after illness or injury. It has been suggested that this might be accomplished through the development of comprehensive rehabilitation programmes. Although in many health and social care organisations a general framework that will or does accommodate rehabilitation provision is emerging, the need for these efforts has become more urgent because of audit commission criticism and the intention to introduce a system of fines where the earlier discharge has not been accommodated by social services.

However, in the management of dependency there is a constant potential impairment at various stages and levels. This causes inappropriate use of scarce and expensive resources and increases the likelihood of waste both in terms of patient or client potential and in the consumption of resources. A suitable intervention which reduces dependency must be available to create a movement towards the rehabilitation of the patient or client so that a natural independence, and if necessary supported independence, is cultivated.

This cannot happen unless there is a continuum of care available which spans the spectrum from acute to community. Below is a checklist for an outline that utilises a variety of techniques including pathways of care for the elderly, programmes of care and care planning and management.

Checklist of techniques that enhance care and release resources

▼ More consideration of the requirements of older people in their recovery from illness and injury, particularly stroke and orthopaedic problems.

▼ Introduction of a multidisciplinary pathway of care team for individual assessment and care management to cover short, medium and longer-term needs, including acute and after care.

▼ Significant steps to unblock beds across the range of service provision through the use, amongst other devices, of partnerships, thereby altering the balance of care in favour of a more appropriate form.

▼ Measures to buy time so that older people experience a reduction in the pressure they now feel to take momentous and sometimes irrevocable decisions regarding their future living arrangements.

▼ Interim arrangements, including comprehensive rehabilitation and follow-up programmes, to enable individuals to make the transition towards greater independence.

▼ Arrangements for management development, monitoring, review and evaluation of programmes.

▼ Identification and redistribution of resources to reflect these movements.

These aspects can be graphically represented so that at various levels of dependency they can be examined and the potential for independence exploited. This is illustrated in Figure 4.8.

Delays in the discharge of older patients can be significantly diminished by tackling the discharge process. This involves the development of close working relationships between external support and the acute sector. The benefits of utilising the potential inherent in adhering to process quality considerations to the full must be emphasised and the need to take control of the process, rather than the process taking control of the circumstances, must always be kept in mind.

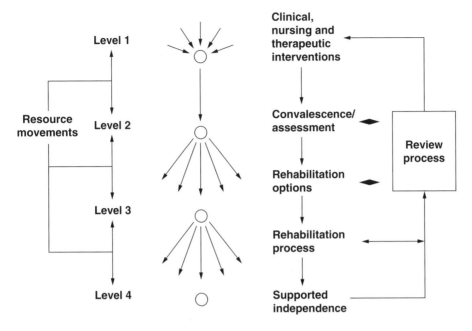

Figure 4.8 Improving independence and re-allocating resources.

Although everyone involved in health and social care must surely desire to accomplish their disparate tasks by doing the right thing at the right time, every time, most are no strangers to the frustrations and limitations that the system can impose. Many of these problems can be alleviated by confronting them directly. Regardless of whether the problems are to do with organisation or with patient or client management, the system or process must be made to serve rather than dominate. Where there is collaboration about the task in hand, benefits both in terms of resources and wellbeing are generated from collaboration and appropriate partnership arrangements.

Tips from the front office

It is important that whilst patient or client needs are pre-eminent, resource implications are not ignored and proper account is taken of any changes. This should in no way be used to slow any improvement or development down as this would clearly be counterproductive. Make sure therefore that:

▼   the pathway team is comprehensive, including the relevant clinicians, therapeutic experts, community workers and key worker

▼ the key worker concept is consistently applied throughout the process

▼ in the case of emergency or for advice, the key worker is available within reason

▼ the patient or client is consulted at every stage and that the options are clearly explained

▼ relatives and carers feel involved in the process

▼ there is a reasonable balance between delay and decision time – delay between stages is minimised but not at the expense of reasonable time being given to the patient or client to decide

▼ patient or client needs come first

▼ there is a continuous awareness of cost, waste and savings

▼ resource implications are properly identified and re-allocations are made on a scientific basis.

Key action points

▼ *The difference between supply and demand* will be reflected in expectation.

▼ *Costs* have to be related to work done in order to be meaningful.

▼ *Budgets* must reflect the cost of workload at an agreed level and standard.

▼ *Comparative costs* do not necessarily compare like with like but they are indicators that may be used to set national tariffs.

▼ Managers must be competent in *interpretation* and in *appropriate intervention* to improve costs.

▼ *Workloads* are affected by changes in dependency.

▼ *Dependency* must be managed at appropriate levels.

5

Managing within time limits

In resource management, it is impossible to ignore the questions:

- Have we got the time to make adjustments or changes?
- Can we buy more time?
- How long will our resources last?
- What was accomplished in a given time?

Time is therefore both a measure of performance and a resource to be managed.

The issues

- All organisations, both public and private, work within an annual time frame for reporting and accounting purposes.
- Therefore as well as being a resource, time is used to measure success.
- Expiring time limits constantly threaten objectives, especially in the context of creating savings.
- Conversely there is always the fear that what has not been used will be forfeited forever.
- The degree of resource mobility is an important factor in development.
- Big numbers must be kept in perspective and large-scale savings plans spread over years.
- In managing larger-scale projects where there is a delay in resource deliveries, expediency sometimes triumphs over caution.
- However, sometimes delay can provide an advantage.

Introduction

As with other more tangible resources, time is always scarce and it is also the key to measuring the rate of resource consumption. These are critical factors in achieving objectives. Compensation for perceived deficiencies can often be made by increasing the number of resources available. However, as the end of a financial period or other deadline approaches and much more work is necessary, a less than cautious approach to the way resources are commissioned and managed can occur.

Escalating demand and expectation of constant improvement require the making of savings in terms of time and money. However, successful managers are able to balance savings and improvements against challenging time frames so that as many as possible of these potential threats are utilised as opportunities.

Despite the allocation of funds that are to be spent on specific purposes and within a defined timescale, most managers have an instinctive drive to accomplish tasks in less time and with less effort, thus creating savings or surpluses. Indeed, the demand for the achievement of more quality activity for less money in a shorter time (QUALMIST) is a phenomenon common to both health and social care.

However, this phenomenon may be prevalent to an unreasonable extent in the upper reaches of an organisation. This is sometimes characterised by constant cuts based upon the assumption that 'they can do what they did last year'. As we shall see, this is a blunt instrument in a sophisticated world. Unfortunately it also generates the growth of a disparate counterproductive subculture which encourages waste by creating demands for more than is needed and a longer timescale (DEMNALTS).

But what are savings or surpluses? Are they, for example, the end products of all those hundreds of efforts to reduce costs that are made daily by diligent, cost-conscious managers? Do we mean the development of better working practices, probably using more modern techniques and technology? Are they the results of major initiatives that involve restructuring, rationalisation and retraction?

Although there is no foreseeable shortage of patient or clients, scarcity of resources needed to cope with this escalating pressure is a persistent and permanent economic phenomenon that has been experienced by managers throughout the ages. Shortage of funds is what comes first to most people's minds, but scarcity in health and social care pervades every type of resource. Below is a checklist of some familiar examples.

Checklist of familiar examples of scarcity in health and social care

▼   Specialist and non-specialist expertise needed to do the evolving tasks that are being constantly revised and refined.

▼   Adequate and safe spaces in which to work.
▼   Sufficient beds or patient/client places to provide proper care.
▼   The right level of care and maintenance to keep equipment in the required functioning mode.
▼   Laundry and linen services provided in the necessary quantities to cope with ever-increasing turnover and higher levels of dependency.
▼   Allowances of time commensurate with safety and security.
▼   Adequate funds and time.

Timing and other factors

Planning, purchasing, commissioning and recruiting take time and training additional specialist professionals can be a much longer process. This is generally referred to as lead time. Where equipment fails unexpectedly or a new development requiring extra resources has been overlooked, a request for exra funding will be more difficult to process if the deadline for the submission of requests has passed.

It is vitally important that managers maintain a keen eye on these so-called lead times and on the progress of new development monies. In order to save unnecessary wastes of time, they must make some advance preparation against the possibility of losing a key resource, the replacement of which is going to be a prolonged affair. Below are some suggestions.

● Major pieces of equipment over £10,000

  – Expect a maximum lifespan of three years, so look out for increasing breakdown and repair.
  – Keep abreast of new developments.
  – Have current sources and up-to-date prices available.
  – Submit your bid at the right time and in anticipation.

● Key professional staff

  – Expect staff to be ambitious, so don't be taken by surprise when someone wants to move on.
  – Be alert to speculation about a staff member's intentions.
  – Know the age structure of the staff, so imminent retirement is not a shock.
  – Have job descriptions ready.

In the course of a year, in addition to these potential delays, the day-to-day resource requirements are not evenly spread. This is due in part to seasonal pressure from patients and clients, for example with winter chest problems, and partly to the need to cope with staff sickness, holidays and weekend arrangements. There are also other factors such as cold weather having an effect upon heating.

Thus determining the rate of consumption is not straightforward and where reductions in the number and scope of resources are required, it can be a tortuous business. This is because there will be elements inside and outside the organisation committed to slowing, if not completely stopping, the process. It is crucial therefore that this phenomenon is clearly understood at all levels of the organisation.

Below is a checklist of some key influences that affect capacity to make major savings.

Key considerations in saving and spending

▼   Sudden availability of spare cash will not be an immediate answer to a vast number of complex problems.

▼   Even if you are fortunate enough to benefit from an extra injection of money, it usually comes earmarked for specific purposes and cannot be used to off-set current overspending.

▼   There is the further complication of apparently unhelpful attitudes in the upper reaches of the organisation where there appears to be an abiding conviction that lower levels have more resources than necessary.

▼   There is the opposite belief at lower levels – that there are insufficient resources to cope with current problems.

▼   Perception of this constant downward pressure to achieve more quality activity for less money in a shorter time (QUALMIST) is complemented by a subculture prevalent at all levels which encourages waste by creating demands for more than is needed (DEMN).

▼   Resource reserves have to be created to cover times in the financial period when demand becomes uneven (e.g. holiday periods, weekends, winter months, etc.).

▼   Remaining resources must be spread out over the weeks, months and year.

▼   If there is going to be a shortfall then the sooner this is detected, the better.

Short-term effects of delay

Delay has two opposing effects on the management of resources. It is frustrating and potentially hazardous when key resources cannot be delivered in time. In these circumstances, correct sourcing and timing are key elements in the commissioning process and managers must take steps to ensure that all possible impediments are removed. Conversely, delay is also the basis of a commonly practised tactic to reduce spending in times of crisis. Halting the painting or building programme, a moratorium on replacement staff or delaying the start of a new development are all recognisable examples of reactions to a shortage of funds. They are in effect devices to buy a little time. But delay in this context must mean exactly that and should not be used indefinitely.

However, if one part of the commissioning process is under the misapprehension that delay is acceptable, whilst in another there is an urgent desire to expedite matters, then effectiveness will be lost. It is important therefore to make clear what deadlines are expected.

The internal demand for resources in any organisation is satisfied through a wide variety of mechanisms. In larger organisations, both purchasing and commissioning are undertaken at a variety of levels and often the individual manager 'on the floor' is unaware of the transaction. The main levels are:

- frontline purchasing of 'raw' resources, including staff
- alternative limited competitive tendering for blocks of resource provision, i.e. facilities management and a reassessment of the mixed economy
- resource distribution, including staff, to meet the internal needs of the organisation
- commissioning individuals or groups to provide comprehensive ranges of service.

These arrangements can be complex but, from a supplies management point of view, the important factor is that from the outset control of the financial and operational consequences is achieved in time to consider alternatives.

Tracking

The exercise of purchase and distribution of resources and services covers the whole spectrum of spending. It includes the purchase of staff, equipment, materials and services. These are constantly consumed by health and social care organisations' internal environments. It is the rate of consumption of a particular item or group that is the dominant factor in the overall cost of the service provided.

However, it is a little understood fact that, as a direct result of intermediate buying managers' (e.g. supplies, personnel, etc.) key strategic position between internal budget managers and the external market place, they significantly influence the level of the budget set later and the time limit on which delivery depends. At the outset therefore it is vital that purchasing managers measure the rates of consumption and likely lead times accurately so that they influence the setting of initial financial and time targets beneficially.

In order to gain control of the spending cycle, it is necessary both to identify clearly the purchasing source and to keep a record of the various stages through which the commissioning episode will pass. It is also important that budgets are managed in such a way that controls events, which can result from an inability to plan, are reduced to manageable proportions. The following checklist summarises the key points to remember.

Checklist of timing improvements

▼ Not only new projects, but assets nearing the end of their useful and cost-effective life, are identified in sufficient time to plan for their replacement or redeployment.

▼ Through this process the supply manager is placed in a more competent position from which to judge how best to allocate financial resources during a particular financial period.

▼ Later events can then be predicted at a specific time and place, and the budget set accordingly.

▼ Provided that existing resources are subjected to the management process, their need for replacement can generally be signalled through an automated mechanism.

▼ This will commence the commissioning cascade, which should terminate with the fulfilment of all the objectives.

▼ The progress of events must be tracked throughout so that comparison with the budget is possible.

▼ Significant deviations from the timescale must be identified so that intervention either in curbing the spending programme or re-allocating financial resources is facilitated.

▼ Sometimes the combined effect of built-in obsolescence, poor financial foresight and long-term implications of cash ebb and flow may characterise an imminent catastrophe (you run out of money or have a windfall).

▼ In the microsystem, although working within delegated authority, budget managers may implement a spending activity on expertise or goods and services at infrequent and perhaps unfortunate intervals so that the matching of income and expenditure has a haphazard and at best fortuitous appearance (you run out of time or you have too much time to spare).

▼   In these cases, the individual manager has to take responsibility for the potential deficit or surplus.

Timing tactical intervention

Variations in budget performance must be kept constantly under review so that significant trends that are likely to compromise a project are established at as early a stage as possible. Tendencies to underspend or overspend can be indicators. From this analysis, appropriate tactical intervention can be determined and the activity can be made to comply with the right timescales.

Managers must ensure that these indicators are not taken out of context:

- financial gain (underspending) = potential failure to meet deadlines
- financial loss (overspending) = poor timing of purchases and requires urgent revision.

Treatment of both types of variation depends on the speed at which resources can either be made available in the case of a delay or mobilised where the budget has been compressed. These conditions are illustrated in Figure 5.1.

In the specific context of project management and in the limited timescale of a stage in the project, variations $t1$ are at risk of being interpreted by a project board, keen to manage resources in the best possible way, as a financial gain or loss, where $t1$ is the time past and $t2$ is the time remaining.

- The most desirable circumstances would therefore be when $t1$ is near the start-up time.
- The limit of a capacity for tactical intervention happens when $t2$ tends to zero. In others words, when the budget manager is made aware of the situation little or no time remains.

Thus a complex supply system seldom performs in accordance with the target in terms of either time or money. However, in most systems there is only limited toleration of variations. They may be regarded as wasteful because of a clear indication of excess or because resource targets are not being fulfilled. Variations in or about the target are therefore important indicators to

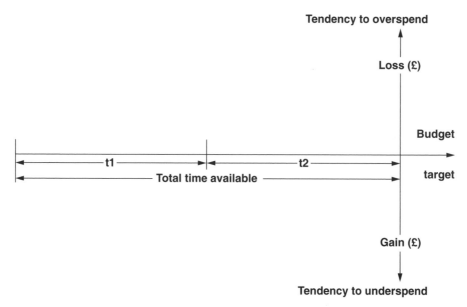

Figure 5.1   Expiring time limit.

performance measured at progressive intervals. Significant factors in relation to these intervals are:

- budget size
- time limit
- completion of the ordering process
- delivery
- payment.

Deviations from the time and budget frame can occur at every one of these levels, as shown in Figure 5.2.

At the point in time where all the commissioning orders have been placed (t1 in the diagram), deliveries (D) will be deliberately behind so that they arrive at the right time and payments will lag further behind. However, in project management analysis this could be regarded as a variation by individual participants. Where it is agreed for one reason or another that deviations are indeed likely, it is important that the remaining time is not tending towards zero when intervention becomes an impossibility.

The single most potent factor in the management of variations is the capacity for beneficial intervention. Intervention is usually necessary to correct both positive and negative deviations so that there is a movement towards that which is perceived to be the normal state. In both cases beneficial intervention is dependent upon:

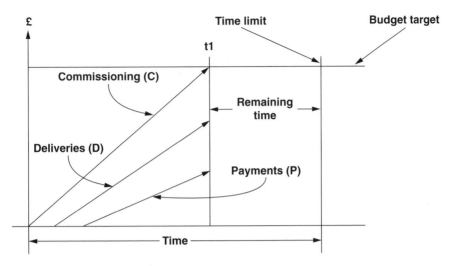

Figure 5.2   Timing tactical intervention.

- rate of fluctuation
- value of the fluctuation
- time available for correction.

A number of attributes are connected with this but, in organisational terms, delay is perhaps the most damaging. Where there is a tendency to over- or underspend, it is essential that supplies managers can take the appropriate action so that variations are constantly under control.

Where it is found that, due to delay factors, budget managers are failing to comply with tolerable limits, acceptability criteria must be tested. Generally, investigations reveal a mixture of causes. Whilst system delays are mainly to blame, a management system must demonstrate punctuality, veracity and simplicity as acceptable characteristics.

Events strings

The simplified string of events which go to make up the commissioning episode is lengthy and the events varied but the major events may be identified as linking supply and spending decisions to fulfilment and actual payment stages. This ensures that everything is counted in. Thus the content of the events diary may be as simple as balancing and reconciling all these factors or it might be made more elaborate, depending on requirements.

Checking the procedures involved in a successful operation provides an extra safeguard for the paymaster function. Apart from the internal security

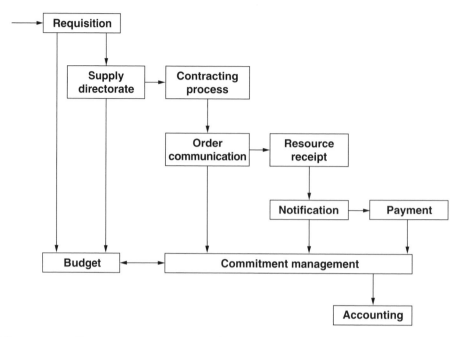

Figure 5.3   Commissioning events trail.

aspect, an improvement in overall financial control will be noted. A simplified form of events trail is illustrated in Figure 5.3.

As suggested at the beginning of this chapter (*see* page 69), managers have to consider alternatives when all or part of a resource package needed to implement a particular stage of development is deficient or cannot be delivered on time, or when a previously agreed budget has to be compressed due to economic pressure.

It is perfectly natural in circumstances where delay potential is prevalent to seek to rectify the emerging situation so that possible time lost is either eliminated or significantly diminished. With a rapidly expiring time limit, a problem occurs between the desire to conform and the obvious increasing need for expediency. However, corrective action is often frustrated by administrative machinery intended to discourage potentially wasteful endeavours and expediency therefore would never be viewed as an efficient device.

Where there is a failure to deliver, an unwelcome by-product is underspending, which in a spending round review might well be mopped up by the project board. The result is that a project manager's response to urgency has to be tempered by caution. Conversely, because of financial constraints, a budget may have to be compressed. This forces a project into an overspending position. Managers need to consider the criteria that must be applied so that expediency in meeting the time target does not impair prospective quality nor adversely affect budget management.

Implementing savings programmes

Programmes for savings can seldom be implemented at the start of a financial period. Below is a checklist of significant factors.

Checklist of factors that cause delay in applying savings

▼   The exact savings amounts may not be known.
▼   Specific areas where savings may be obtained take time to identify.
▼   Consultation, if this is necessary, may take time.
▼   Methods for implementation may be obstructed, for example consultation or some other impediment may not have been properly contemplated.
▼   Implementation may prove more difficult than anticipated.

As the time limit expires, the potential for realising the full target will not be achieved until the next or subsequent financial period. This is illustrated in Figure 5.4.

Within a limited timescale a lack of compliance at t1 is at risk of being misinterpreted as a financial gain or loss. The situation in Figure 5.1 is repeated.

●   The most desirable circumstances would therefore be when t1 is near the start-up time.
●   The limit of a capacity for any savings is when t2 tends to zero.

In others words, when the budget manager is made aware of the situation little or no time remains.

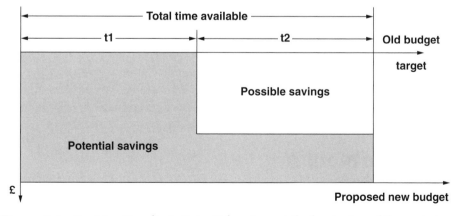

Figure 5.4   Expiring time limit. Potential savings at the beginning of the period are gradually reduced to possible savings as time progresses.

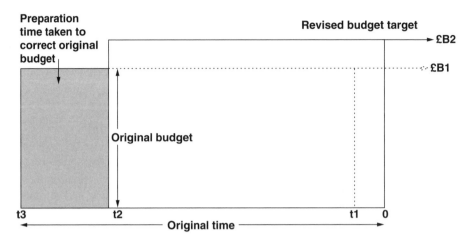

Figure 5.5   Establishing the financial episode.

When allocations of time and money are received, account has also to be taken of the fact that although these resources should represent a certain level of commissioning power, because of the marginal activity mentioned earlier and other factors, this strict relationship may not be maintained. The manager must inevitably have regard to this situation and through it, attempt effective management.

At the outset therefore it is important that the right time frame and the correct budget are allocated. This involves taking up some of the time to assess the exact financial consequences. This process is illustrated in Figure 5.5.

The limiting situations are as follows:

- at t3 the original time span within which the task was to be completed is at its maximum but the estimated budget B1 is too low
- at t2, following fuller research, quotations, etc. a revised higher budget B2 has been allocated together with an extension of the time limit
- between t2 and zero (the expiry of the time limit) a firm commitment to purchase or release resources must be made so that the objectives may be met; also during this time, efforts must be made to ensure that either the two objectives are met or an alternative is found
- at zero there must be a reconciliation between budget and achievement.

Resource mobility

Timing is therefore a key element in measuring performance and resource mobility, availability and the achievement of tasks. In determining resource mobility, the following limits must be established.

- *Developments*. Where managers are trying to improve services, they must ensure that the resources they need can be made available within the time frame. Thus if the delivery time, start time or lead time is greater than the time allowed in the business plan, then achievement of the proposal will fail.
- *Retraction*. Where there has to be a rationalisation of resources, a consequent budget reduction and redistribution of funds will be dependent on the achievement of objectives within the time frame. Where costs are of a continuous nature, like payroll, rentals and other contractual obligations, these will continue to mount up until a suitable form of intervention is activated.
- *Availability in development*. The availability of resources needed to develop or sustain a service within a time limit can be written as

$$Av = t$$

where Av is availability and t is the expiring time limit. If the time limit is expiring, the availability will be zero, the business planning test will be negative and the proposal in that form will fail. However, success will prevail as long as the remaining time is greater than zero.
- *Mobility in retraction*. In order to meet the savings targets imposed by a rationalisation situation, it is sensible to ensure that the mobility of resources intended for decommissioning at any time is greater than the saving required. For example, if the saving required is S, the resource mobility factor, Rm, should always exceed this.

$$Rm > S$$

As time expires, this mobility factor has to increase proportionately. Thus at an expiry time t, S is taken to be constant and the equation can be written,

$$Rmt = S$$

Therefore where t is very small, Rm would have to become increasingly manageable – where $t \rightarrow 0$, $Rm \rightarrow \infty$ which would be clearly impossible.

The converse of this also applies and released resources can be reallocated to developments but not usually on the same scale. The problem is the difficulty involved in introducing a spending regime which would conform to the principles outlined. For example, if a business plan proposes service developments in the order of £4 million, dependent upon a rationalisation plan of similar dimensions, it is unlikely than the two programmes could coexist completely within the same time frame because as soon as the clock started to run $t \rightarrow 0$.

Timing is therefore a key element in measuring resource mobility, availability and the achievement of tasks. Where it is found that due to delay factors, project managers are failing to comply with tolerable limits, acceptability criteria must be tested. Generally, investigations reveal a mixture of three causes. Whilst it might be that system delays are mainly to blame, there may also be confusion on the part of the budget manager, firstly in believing the results and secondly in interpreting them correctly. In order to obtain the time spans necessary for successful intervention, a system must therefore demonstrate punctuality, veracity and simplicity as acceptable characteristics. The following key points have to be borne in mind.

- Increasing mobility and availability can be obtained by reducing the potential lifespan of resources through greater dependence on leasing, the employment of temporary staff, overtime, etc.
- However, in the rationalisation situation a critical mobility mass may develop.
- Similarly, in a development situation, where the desired resources have a long delivery lead, the capability of the business plan may be impaired.
- In both cases there can be loss of morale, increases in sickness levels, diminished performance, greater staff turnover and a marked unwillingness on the part of staff to accept a post within the organisation.
- This turbulence will be potentially destructive and compares unfavourably with the more dynamic organisation.
- Critical mobility mass often occurs before the final stages of a change.

Tip from the front office

In stabilising existing services or where an alteration in the balance of care is required, the quality, consumption, availability and mobility of the resources used to support these services are key factors in creating and managing the movement needed to accommodate service change and improvement.

Big numbers in perspective

Out of context, making £1 million of savings seems an unreasonable objective. If your annual budget is around £1 million, then there would be some substance to your reservations – unless, of course, you were prepared to think the unthinkable! However, spread it over a number of years and the cumulative effect is amazing. For example, if you were able to save £10,000 on a cumulative basis every year for ten years, you would have saved £550,000 at the end of the period.

This is the reverse application of the system much favoured in recent years by the chancellor, who wishes to make the most of monies he is proposing to make available in succeeding years. It is the result of applying a well-known arithmetic series formula. The series in this case is 10, 20, 30, 40, 50, 60, 70, 80, 90, 100. To obtain the total of all the numbers in the series, add the first number in the series (10) to the last number in the series (100), divide by two (to obtain the average) and multiply by the number in the series:

$$10 + 100 = 110$$

$$\frac{110}{2} = 55$$

$$55 \times 10 = 550$$

It is interesting to note that although the savings total £550,000, over the period of time the budget would only have been reduced by £100,000.

Of course, unless the budget of £1 million represents a service that is to be discontinued or some other radical solution is being applied, for example the loss of a contract to an outside contractor, it unlikely that such a disproportionately large amount of savings would be expected or that such a long period would be agreed.

Budgets in the order of £20–50 million are more realistic vehicles for targets of this magnitude but it is imperative that managers put the potential for saving into perspective. This means that the time frame for achievement has to be realistic and the savings therefore spread over a number of years, although ten is somewhat extreme.

Key action points

▼ It is essential that managers keep the best interests of patients and clients constantly in mind and do not become distracted by other pressures.

▼ Funding problems on a fairly large scale will continue to be reflected in limited resource availability and within well-defined time limits.

▼ Further complications arise when managers need to adapt to clinical and other developments and find themselves limited by time and resources.

▼ There are no easy or quick solutions but approaching the problem over a period of time will get results.

▼ Significant savings can be made from already overstretched resources by better understanding and comprehension and by bidding for more time in the same way as with other resources.

▼ Big number budget reductions are prevailing factors.

▼ In order to make progress, there must be unity of purpose at all levels of the organisation.

▼ Large-scale savings have to be broken down into manageable components.

▼ The time available to make savings is a critical consideration.

▼ Time frames have to be reasonable.

▼ Timing has to be high on the management agenda for consultation and negotiation.

6

Commissioning resources

Appropriate and effective purchasing or commissioning of resources is crucial to quality and performance. However, because it is so specialised, often technical and frequently undertaken at a distance, managers have a tendency to leave the detail to the 'experts'. This can lead to mistakes, coupled with communication problems, that result in wasteful practices.

The issues

- It is the objective of all purchasing and commissioning to obtain goods and services at the right time and right price, in the right quantity and at the right quality.
- This is mainly managed by the regulation of fair and appropriate competition.
- Resource purchasing or commissioning is undertaken on behalf of frontline managers by specialists (personnel, supplies, pharmacy, works, etc.).
- However, authority and responsibility continue to reside with the individual manager who creates the demand.
- The lines of responsibility and communication must be clear.
- Specifications, priorities and prioritisation must be agreed by the individual manager.
- Managers must participate in supply chain management and properly 'sign off' goods and services once they are satisfied that they conform with expectation.

Introduction

Value for money is the essence of purchasing and commissioning. This is normally obtained through the testing of the market for a particular item by open, fair and appropriate competition. But markets are seldom homogeneous in nature, nor can their size and scope be limited by artificial boundaries. However, it is possible to obtain a feeling for the way in which markets operate by ignoring these complications and assuming that there is equality.

From the commissioner's or purchaser's point of view, the importance of purchasing power can never be overemphasised. Clearly operators who can command global markets and whose contracts are on that scale have a significant advantage over smaller-scale purchasers and are able to use their purchasing power to drive down prices. It is for this reason that contracting is located as far up the organisational scale as possible, standardisation is to be greatly encouraged and, where possible, government departments and other structures share some of the common purchasing resources, for example HM Stationery Office.

Where no regulation prohibits, there is therefore a tendency to form alliances or consortia in both purchaser/commissioner and supplier modes whilst at the same time encouraging the mixed economy of care. These groupings are called 'strategic alliances.' In commercial practice, this concept is further extended to include the suppliers so that they are locked more permanently into the supply chain.

Although these factors are important contradictory influences in commercial buying and selling and they must be borne in mind, in health and social care it is usual to obtain the best result from a mixture of applications because of the enormous range of goods and services purchased. Thus an alliance that has been temporarily formed by two trusts, for example, may have a sceptical reception from service commissioners. However, the benefits of cost effectiveness and value for money of such proposals, together with the suggested improvements in the quality of patient/client care, would be attractive.

In large-scale purchasing, the formality and methods used to achieve value for money vary according to the type and size of the prospective purchase. For example, the way we recruit staff is obviously different to the method used to buy a pencil and this in turn differs from purchases of drugs or x-ray equipment. And in the same way, each broad category requires the dedication of different types of professional service. In other words, the methods used to purchase goods and services vary according to their:

- *Type*. Whether they fall broadly into the various resource categories already identified (i.e. staffing, estate, medical equipment, drugs or other supplies) will determine the professional agency that will process the request.
- *Size*. The size or other requirement (e.g. safety, cold rooms or ventilation) of the item could pose a problem and may involve other professionals.

- *Value.* If the value is small, a less formal tendering and contracting arrangement may be made.
- *Volume or security.* Where volumes are large (e.g. disposable items) or where there is a specific security requirement (e.g. drugs), interim storage with special facilities may be needed.

Purchasing/commissioning options

In health and social care organisations, the urgency with which many of the resources are required has to be neatly balanced with both the ability to pay and the absolute need to render a proper account of just how they were obtained. Whilst this gives a degree of flexibility, the connection between these three facets can never be ignored.

The actual acts of purchasing and commissioning are key to the efficient and effective management of resources, which must be apparent and transparent, and are the responsibility of specialist purchasing agents or directorates, such as personnel, supplies, works, pharmacy, etc. The determination of their roles is the result of fairly complex rules, routes and structures peculiar to the particular needs of the individual health or social care organisation. In order to conform with the need for fiscal rectitude, it is important that all staff recognise and accept this position and are never tempted into a situation where they believe that they are empowered to undertake any of these tasks, no matter how much they know about particular equipment, drugs or any other resources.

Conversely, it is equally important that those whose job it is to carry out the acts of procurement realise that they act on behalf of the individual manager who has the authority to make the request and that the two parties must work harmoniously together to acquire best value for money. Where there is any doubt, the correct lines of communication must be defined.

The concept of the branches of a tree illustrates the way in which the wide spectrum of resource consumption has to be integrated with purchasing sources or directorates. In Figure 6.1 the relationship between the main purchasing agents or directorates emphasises the extremely specialised and professional nature of resource procurement.

Where a large-scale purchase is contemplated, a building project is to be undertaken, a service is to be subjected to a contracting out process or where patient/client services are to be sought outside the organisation, more complex arrangements which involve a wide spectrum of interested parties will be required.

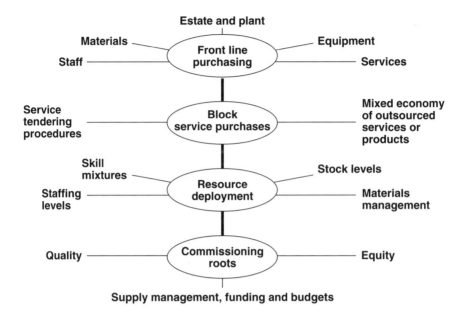

Figure 6.1   The supply tree branches.

In all cases a wide range of purchasing/commissioning options is available. The guiding principle in all cases is to minimise bureaucracy and actual cost of purchasing, whilst at the same time maintaining standards. The main options are summarised in the checklist below.

Checklist of purchasing/commissioning options

▼   *Make.* In almost all health and social care organisations there is a degree of 'industrial productivity', which ranges from generating heat and sometimes power, to processing laundry, CSSD and perhaps specialised sterile fluids. In addition, large-scale photocopying and computerised form production are commonplace. The question of whether an item could or should be made on site or nearby is always worth considering.

▼   *Hire.* Where the requirement is once only or at most very infrequent, the hire of premises, equipment, transport or specialised services is an important purchasing device, which avoids longer-term commitment and lack of resource mobility. However, the number of times that this occurs must be kept under review so that use of the option is always shown to be cost effective and good value for money.

▼ *Rent*. Rental agreements are longer-term commitments and avoid the use of capital monies and charges. The automatic replacement with new equipment also maintains the developmental spectrum and reduces the overall cost of repairs.

▼ *Directly employ*. Various options that regulate the hiring of staff are constantly being examined and more flexible arrangements that have mutual benefits are key to successful labour relations.

▼ *Buy*. Depending on the volume and size of the proposed purchase or commission, the act of buying will be subject to:

- an on-the-spot purchase where the item is small, probably from petty cash
- the best value for money out of three quotations, where the purchases are small in either volume and/or cost
- for similar minor purchases, a repeat order may be issued where the price and quality have been guaranteed
- for larger items or where the number of small items is large, more formal procedures involving invitations to tender from competent contractors will be invoked (this is dealt with in the section starting on page 110)
- off-contract purchases are and should be able to carry the main volume of purchases. The contracts themselves may be arranged either centrally, regionally or locally depending on the type and volume of the particular goods and services required.

▼ *Share*. The decision to share a resource purchase with another authority or trust will be taken on the grounds of utility and overall benefit. It also includes the possibility of entering into a more formal partnership agreement or arrangement and this has been extended to include partnerships that pertain to the care of patients/clients such as the older patient. This is dealt with in Chapter 8.

▼ *Contract out*. This occurs where large and easily identifiable portions of an organisation, such as catering, cleaning, portering, laundry services, etc. can be subjected to a competitive tendering process to determine the best way of providing these services. Further information is provided in the section starting on page 110.

▼ *Rationalise service*. In extreme cases, for example where a building or a service is discovered to be on the point of collapse, a service rationalisation may be needed instead of further investment.

▼ *Do nothing*. This is always an option that should be considered, but the question 'What would happen if ... ?' should be answered by the manager, not the agent.

Tips from the front office

In order to commission high-quality patient/client care, we must

- identify and prioritise demands
- focus on the needs of the patient/client
- integrate or rationalise care or treatment so that it is effective
- make the best possible use of scarce resources
- accept responsibility and facilitate accountability.

We must constantly ask ourselves the questions

- shall we diversify, specialise or stay the same?
- shall we expand, contract or maintain the status quo?

Acceptability criteria

Acceptability criteria for the acquisition of resources are important to resource managers for two reasons. First, they are the broad indicators that match health and social care organisations with suitably competent contractors and secondly, they are important where a resource manager is required to submit an in-house tender for contracting out purposes. It is therefore a good discipline to check whether the individual manager can meet all criteria whilst developing and implementing such criteria for purchases from external sources.

In commissioning resources from an external source, all parties must be clear about the potential contractor's ability to satisfy in all respects the health and/or social care organisation's requirements and culture (provided this is not exclusive). For example, to be considered competent to satisfy the potentially vast demands placed upon them, contractors must be able to demonstrate their track record and show that they are capable of delivering the range of facilities in the volumes specified and within the timescales indicated. They must have satisfactory staffing with the right qualifications, experience and structures, and have a reputation for fair employment policies. In addition, where health and social care organisations are committed to a particular ethical or moral position, for example a rejection of the smoking habit or global fair trade, potential contractors would have to conform in the most obvious respects so that there would be no future embarrassment. Conflicts of interest could also be prejudicial. Below is a checklist of the main acceptability criteria that need to be considered.

Checklist of acceptability criteria for competent contractors

▼ *Capability.* Competent contractors can show that they have the capability to adhere in all respects to the physical conditions such as making a quality product or, in the case of patient/client care, have the ability to provide the quality services required.

▼ *Capacity.* To be considered, they have to show that they are a big enough organisation to handle the volumes at the stated price and deliver to the requisite destinations in the times and frequency stipulated.

▼ *Conflict of interest.* Competent contractors should have no conflict of interest that is prejudicial to fair dealing or transparent contracting. They should never be in a position where they can influence the course of the tendering or contract process.

▼ *Reputation.* Their reputation as a producer or provider of a service has to be acceptable and generally they must show, by means of references to work previously undertaken, that their record is satisfactory.

▼ *Regulation and legislation.* Contractors must show that they conform in all respects to regulations that govern the way their organisation performs.

▼ *Staffing structure and policy.* A competent contractor will be able and delighted to demonstrate that their internal organisation adequately supports the tasks required and that they operate staffing policies that are commensurate with those required by health and social care organisations.

▼ *Qualifications.* In complex contracts, particularly in contracting out and in commissioning patient/client services, the requisite levels of staff competence will have to be demonstrated.

▼ *Sub-contracting.* In large contracts, most health and social care organisations will want to know whether there will be an element of sharing or out-sourcing and if that is the position they may wish to ensure that all the above requirements are replicated by the subcontractor.

▼ *Ethical or moral considerations.* Competent contractors are generally expected to conform with any agreed codes of conduct or ethical positions adopted by heath and social care organisations.

▼ *Audit or other types of inspection.* Contractors and health and social care organisations must agree upon the method for ensuring consistent compliance with all the conditions listed if the contract is awarded.

Resource commissioning process

As stated above, in the context of commissioning, resource managers must be constantly alert to the viability, cost effectiveness and relative quality of the service they provide, particularly where large-scale out-sourcing or competitive tender is contemplated. While they are engaged in the specification process, they should constantly check their performance against that which they are specifying for an external provider. For guidance, a broad outline of an integrated commissioning/internal improvement process, which can include patient/client services and contracting out, is shown in Figure 6.2.

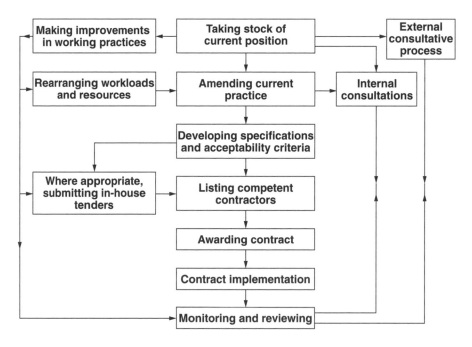

Figure 6.2   Integrated commissioning.

In Figure 6.2, individual resource managers are shown to be shadowing the commissioning process in order to ensure compliance with service requirements. However, where they were expected to submit an in-house tender, they would be excluded from direct input into the process so that they too could demonstrate that there was no conflict of interest.

Internal and external consultation is very important where large-scale contracts are contemplated.

Below is a checklist of important points.

Checklist of main points for commissioning resources and services

Resource managers must be involved at all stages in the commissioning/ purchasing process. The main points to remember are:

▼   *User requirements, sourcing supplies and specifications*
  – examine volumes and move towards appropriate standardisation
  – simplify and rationalise the number of similar items in speci-
    fications.
▼   *Evaluate purchasing power and identify strategic alliances.* Examine
  options to increase purchasing power through partnership or agency
  arrangements with other purchasing organisations.
▼   *Develop corporate policy on contingency requirements*
  – ensure flexibility in contract arrangements
  – delegate more purchasing to local level
  – look at vertical integration and just-in-time (JIT) policies.
▼   *Choose competent contractors* who can guarantee supplies and have an
  established reputation. Check out the nature of their assurances.
▼   *Post-tender negotiations.* It is sometimes considered appropriate to
  follow up the receipt of tenders with briefing or debriefing sessions
  when further considerations and more details are discussed and
  agreed; these can include concerns over deliveries.
▼   *Review facilities* for the reception and storage of goods and services.
▼   *Constantly review* contingency reserves through adequate audit and
  other systems.

Until recently no threat or interruption of supplies was perceived in the modern world of commerce and supply lines were often tortuously long. Although reserve stocks and stockpiling are still regarded as wasteful and there is still heavy reliance on just-in-time deliveries, recent petrol delivery crises, the threat of terrorist disruption on a large scale and the realisation following the foot-and-mouth crisis that food is often transported over incredible distances to reach the consumer have made the government and managers think again. Nevertheless, resource managers need to bear in mind the *Don'ts* in the checklist overleaf.

Checklist of stockpile do's and don'ts

▼   Don't stockpile – it eats up cash and causes waste.
▼   Do keep stocks to a minimum.
▼   Overstocking provides temptation to the potential pilferer.
▼   Don't waste energy and time on hostility to stock initiatives with unattractive objectives.
▼   Don't economise at the expense of health and safety.
▼   Don't ignore complaints or warnings about potential hazards.
▼   Don't make unnecessary risks.
▼   Don't allow materials to become out of date.

Tips from the front office

▼   Increased volume can often be obtained at an agreed cost.
▼   Limited volume can mask underutilised resources.
▼   Low volumes can be a threat to safety due to lack of practice.
▼   High volumes may also be unsafe because of overwork.
▼   Plan for adequate contingencies.
▼   Ensure shelf lives of contingency supplies are appropriate.
▼   Contingency stock movements should comply with usual in and out flow.
▼   Quality is compliance with the appropriate specification; it is *not* usually the most expensive item.
▼   Quantities should always be exact. Make sure that you are using the correct unit, i.e. one only, tens, dozens, hundreds, gross, etc.
▼   Check out the efficacy of just-in-time stock management systems.
▼   Where stocks are maintained at low levels, timely deliveries are essential.

Intangible benefits

Where there are options in terms of the feasibility of a proposal, the method used to purchase or commission (rent or buy, etc.) or the choice of contractor, there are usually a number of intangible benefits to be considered. Unless some rational system for considering them is accepted by the commissioning group, it will be impossible to arrive at a coherent decision. Below is a checklist of suggested steps for achieving consensus.

Checklist of intangible benefit considerations

▼ List all the expected benefits, for example quality, accessibility, ease of introduction, whether the proposal is in keeping with strategic objectives, etc.
▼ Give each expected benefit a rating or score out of 100. This is called the weighting.
▼ Separately, give a score for each of the expected benefits as delivered by each tender.
▼ Then multiply each benefit score by the relevant weighting.
▼ Add the benefit scores to give a total for each tender.
▼ Pick out the tender which gives the most benefit from the totals line.
▼ If this is not the cheapest tender further consideration is required, for example, how close the cheapest tender is to the one which delivers the most intangible benefits.

An example of this type of exercise is illustrated in the case study below.

Case study

St Bedeful Trust received five tenders for the replacement of x-ray equipment. One was approximately 50% more than the prices quoted by the other four and was for a make of equipment unknown to the panel. That tender was therefore disqualified on the grounds of price. As the other four tenders were relatively close in terms of price, but offered different types of support or other benefits (such as capacity), the panel decided to weigh up the benefits.

In addition to their already developed acceptability criteria, they added speed of delivery, ease of installation, guarantees, call out and defective replacement facilities, and other quality issues. The weighting they attributed to each is shown in Table 6.1; their subsequent analyses are shown in Tables 6.2 and 6.3.

Table 6.1 Intangible benefit criteria and weighting

Detail	Weighting
Speed of delivey	30
Ease of installation (disruption factor)	20
Guarantees	20
Response times and distances in case of a fault	10
Acceptability criteria	10
Other quality issues	10
Total	100

In Table 6.2 tender 2 has the highest score.

Table 6.2 Scores for each tender

Detail	Tender 1	Tender 2	Tender 3	Tender 4
Speed of delivery	7	9	10	8
Ease of installation (disruption factor)	7	9	10	8
Guarantees	5	9	9	6
Response times and distances in case of a fault	6	8	9	5
Acceptability criteria	5	6	5	5
Other quality issues	4	8	5	5
Total	34	49	48	37

However, in Table 6.3 tender 3 has the highest weighted benefit.

Table 6.3 Weighted benefit (multiplies values in Table 6.2 with those in Table 6.1)

Detail	Tender 1	Tender 2	Tender 3	Tender 4
Speed of delivery	210	270	300	240
Ease of installation (disruption factor)	140	180	200	160
Guarantees	100	180	180	120
Response times and distances in case of a fault	60	80	90	50
Acceptability criteria	50	60	50	50
Other quality issues	40	80	50	50
Total	600	850	870	670

Tips from the front office

▼   Where an option has the lowest cost but is the least beneficial, it will be eliminated.
▼   Conversely, where an option is the most preferred option but it is also the most costly, a further process is necessary.
▼   This will have to take the sensitivity of service requirements into account.
▼   If cost differentials turn out to be small, the favoured option might still succeed.

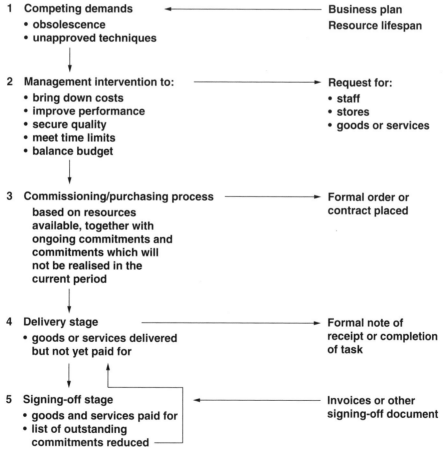

Figure 6.3   Commissioning stages.

Tips from the front office

▼   Always make sure that there is appropriate documentation to cover any agreement.
▼   Never negotiate an external contract without proper professional help.
▼   Make sure that the financial arrangements have been properly endorsed.
▼   Don't provide any services until customers have indicated their understanding of the terms of the agreement.
▼   After delivery, don't let contractors leave without ensuring that their financial obligations have been discharged also.

Where goods and services are delivered direct to the department managers, they should:

▼   make sure that they have the correct copy of the buying order
▼   tell accounts staff if goods do not turn up at the expected time because this might be because they have been lost in transit and this may render the organisation liable
▼   check all details immediately on receipt
▼   where there is a discrepancy, inform the relevant party without delay
▼   sign and return all documents to the accounts department expeditiously.

Case study

St Bedeful Trust, Smalltown Trust and Bigtown Social Services entered an ambitious partnership arrangement aimed at providing a seamless service for the following:

●   an assessment and rehabilitation unit for older and disabled patients/clients
●   short-term respite care facilities for community carers
●   community support through the establishment of pathways of care teams.

The joint project was to be based in the vacant accommodation at Smalltown Infirmary which required remedial works to cope with its change of use. The joint project board set aside some funds to cover a number of key interface areas and these are shown in Table 6.4.

Table 6.4 Estimated cost of proposed developments

Joint project: proposed developments	Cost (£k)
Capital cost of refurbishing and commissioning 'new' accommodation at Smalltown Infirmary to provide assessment, rehabilitation and respite facilities	500
Revenue cost of care in assessment unit development	560
Revenue cost of rehabilitation (daily living, etc.)	120
Additional revenue costs of a multidisciplinary pathway of care team for individual assessment and care management to cover short, medium and longer-term needs, including acute and after care	57
Additional cost of comprehensive rehabilitation and follow-up programmes to enable individuals to make the transition towards greater independence	47
Additional cost of arrangements for management development, monitoring, review and evaluation of programmes	50
Total	1334

Key action points

▼ Value for money is a key principle in commissioning resources.

▼ It is vital to adequately identify and evaluate the quantity, quality and nature of internal demand.

▼ Structured tracking procedures from the issue of order communications to receipt and payment must be implemented.

▼ This operation must include all the likely interim events so that amendments and adjustments can be facilitated.

▼ As the episode progresses, timely tactical or strategic intervention to defer or replace a particular item(s) will ensure better supply chain management.

7

Budgets and resources

Budgetary management is a critical measurement of resource performance and an indicator of the need for appropriate intervention. It also gives an important insight into the affordability of the service provided and is a significant indicator of the need to reallocate resources. However, its effectiveness can be impaired because of flaws in organisational, structural or other management arrangements.

The issues

Budget systems are intended as aids to the management of resources. They are not devices for the persecution of managers. Effective budget management systems are governed by a number of factors.

- They must relate costs to budgetary management.
- They must clearly connect income with expenditure.
- They must work within the spending cycle (the financial year) so that accounting and budgetary information can be easily connected.
- The methods used to calculate budgets must be transparent.
- The mechanism should make use of the control points characterised by the various events in the supply chain.
- Variations at each stage must be identified and an appropriate intervention stategy applied.
- Significant and consistent trends usually signal the need to reallocate resources.
- There must be clear accountability.
- The way in which the organisation operates can impair the overall performance of the system.

Introduction

In order to develop and sustain a budget management system, communication at all levels in health and social care organisations is essential. The overall purpose is to assist managers in their pursuit of effective resource usage. But the initiative to make changes should lie with the manager and the subsequent financial report should be the record of that action. This is not a process that tells budget managers from the top down in a one-way dialogue. *Successful budget management systems have two-way communication.*

However, the structure of the organisation may be an inhibiting factor. For example, if the organisation cannot make up its mind between professional and functional lines of financial responsibility, budgetary management in an already complicated arrangement can become confusing. In complex organisations, sometimes apparently contradictory rules have to apply.

The issue of delegated spending authority can therefore be a problem. Although an organisation might desire to make managers responsible, the authority to spend money could be more difficult to relinquish because the bureaucratic instinct is to make so many rules that a budget manager cannot truly exercise fully delegated authority. For example, if a budget manager wants to recruit staff to fill vacancies, it can happen that the personnel department will not accept such a request unless it conforms with other establishment rules. This duplication is wasteful and will inevitably lead to a loss of momentum.

The process of producing budget statements needs to go beyond the simple assembly of facts and figures and must convey the need for budget managers to take remedial action. Clarity, timing, focus, action and reaction are the objectives of good financial communication.

To make this two-way communication more effective, skills in managing within the budgetary environment must also be developed. Enhanced interpretative and intervention capacity is key to improved performance.

What is a budget?

A budget can be defined in financial terms or it can simply be a number or group of resources (e.g. so many staff, an inventory of equipment, a list of permitted rations, etc.), or it can be a combination of both. Managers who receive budgets must know the purposes for which the budgets are intended and any supplementary rules about how the expenditure is to be incurred. Budget managers must also have a clear idea of the timespan that the budget must cover. There are two aspects to this. First, where a budget is for continuous expenditure, like payroll for example, it must be divided out over the number of weeks or months that are in the period so that it can be observed to last out. If however, the budget is for a once-and-for-all project, it usually does not much matter when the budget is exhausted as long as it is spent within the time frame, unless there are other factors to consider. Below is a short definition.

A budget is a set amount of money or a ration of resources allocated to an authorised manager for a specific purpose and intended to cover a defined period of time.

A number of different methods are used for calculating a budget. Below is a checklist of the main methods.

Checklist of princial methods used to calculate or set a budget

▼ *Incremental budgets.* In this case historical expenditure patterns are taken to represent the normal situation and increases due to inflation, together with service developments and cost improvements, are added or subtracted in accordance with agreed planning parameters.

▼ *Zero-based budgets.* These are at the other extreme to incrementalism and involve a complex and radical approach in which baselines are in effect reduced to zero. The budget is built from this position purely on the basis of justified bids. Although at first sight this might seem alien to the public sector, it is in fact prevalent where proposals for capital and non-recurring revenue are concerned. In the case of major expenditure proposals, an option appraisal technique is applied in order to provide a structure for scrutiny and a system of project management is usually applied to ensure compliance with objectives. In these circumstances, the time frame and subsequently the financial consequences will extend beyond the normal one-year limit which is generally applied to other types of expenditure.

▼ *Standards costed budgets.* These occur in more sophisticated approaches to budgets. The technique involves the precise definition of the quality standards which have been agreed and these are then subjected to the precise costing of every item. Budgets are then built up to arrive at an overall cost. The technique has been used increasingly extensively, particularly where a national tariff is contemplated, and implies the introduction of reporting and monitoring arrangements which support the system. It appears logical that these standards are closely linked to cost and price, as discussed in Chapter 3. If this were not so, it is difficult to see how expectations can be realised in a structured way.

▼ *Usage.* Generally speaking, most budget systems make use of different aspects of the above techniques. Where historical baselines have been used and augmented through allowances for inflation, there is a reflection of the incremental approach to budgeting but tempered by a form of cash limits which have been applied to the forecast for inflation. If no other influences were at work, health and social care organisations would be free to find the necessary funding from existing resourcing. On the other hand, where there is a pressure to take quality initiatives, for example in order to conform with charter standards, then there would be internal difficulties in arriving at satisfactory budgets. To compensate, the organisation and the budget manager will have to ensure that the core values for quality reflect the criteria which are previously set out. This is particularly relevant in the application of process quality techniques. Although this application will have the effect of driving down costs, the setting of a budget target must bear a clear relationship to the determining cost.

Budget management system characteristics

It has already been demonstrated that the potential for uncontrolled decision-taking, which can outstrip both expenditure and resources, exists. The latent inevitability about some aspects of expenditure which are the legacy of previous decisions also exists.

The developing information base which coordinates and controls this tripartite interface is set out in the checklist below.

Checklist of coordination and control aspects

The three main facets of budgetary management are:

▼ *facilitate managers in*

  − controlling tasks and costs within known limits
  − deciding which task options must have priority
  − monitoring commitments against expenditure patterns
  − selecting other options where delivery times cannot be met
  − achieving better commissioning and distribution targets
  − rendering improved accountability

▼ *improving overall management which will*

- provide an overview of the total position
- help manage tasks and costs
- facilitate instant monitoring
- show where and when intervention should take place
- indicate areas where resource redistribution can take place

▼ *assist the organisation as a whole in*

- determining the scope of business in financial and other terms
- accessing information on potential business transacted elsewhere
- managing workloads vs. expectation
- measuring performance against known targets
- helping managers to control expenditure within budget limits
- improving total accountability.

There are a number of desirable attributes which an effective budget management system manifests. The main points which must be considered are set out in the checklist below.

Checklist of desirable budget communication attributes

▼ *Clarity*

- active participation in financial planning
- concentration upon fact
- familiarity with terminology.

▼ *Timing*

- curtailing potential losses in transmission
- careful evaluation
- effective intervention.

▼ *Focus*

- valuing income sources
- targeting significant variations
- improving performance.

▼ *Action*

- compliance with business plan
- creating enabling structure

- action planning
- communication audit.

▼   *Reaction*

- diminishing turbulence
- containing any latent hostility
- facilitating the management of change.

Arising from the identification of desirable attributes, budget management statements need to be amenable to easy interpretation and be clear indicators of what has to happen next. Below is a checklist of the main points for consideration.

Checklist for budget document design and interpretation

▼   *Simplicity*

- Documentation flowing from financial regimes must comply with quality and quantity standards.
- In order to reduce frustration at budget-manager level they should be easily interpreted.
- This means that they must be in a language which clearly conveys the meaning.
- Finance staff become accustomed to the use of codes which are alphanumeric in character and there is a temptation not to convert these into terms which can be easily understood by all.
- In this way, a budget manager may be presented with descriptions which are not meaningful.
- Budget reports may also be issued in computer printout form. Some have argued that this can add authority to the document, but it must be considered as unacceptable for the budget manager.
- However, oversimplification of a combination of various disparate elements is to be discouraged. For example, where a number of subgroups are fluctuating in different directions.

▼   *Veracity*

- The initial reaction of most managers, when confronted with disadvantageous figures, is to challenge their accuracy.
- If they are successful in using this tactic, they may gain time and may in the long run escape having to account for their position.

- This avoidance is in nobody's best interest because the long-term damage to the control system and the organisation may be significant.
- It is important therefore that the production of finance information is capable of verification and conveys the true position.

▼ *Punctuality*

- The timing of budget planning, the setting of the budget and the dissemination of budget reports are crucial to the success of the system.
- The main thrust of any budgetary initiative must be the main-tenance of a connection between the objectives, management action and the results. Where a significant gap occurs at any of these stages, controlling influences are diminished and the sys-tem may be relegated to the category of being of historical interest only.
- There are a number of methods which may be used to improve the tenuousness of budgetary information.

▼ *Credibility*

- It is clear that compliance with the three factors, simplicity, verac-ity and punctuality maintains and improves a system's credibility.
- Conversely, dissatisfaction with any, some or all factors may be damaging unless some effort is made to repair the situation.
- However, another more subtle influence lies in the determination of managers and management to take action on the information provided.
- If there is an indication that a significant variation is developing and no corrective action is taken, it could be argued that, by default, credibility is impaired.
- It is important therefore that acceptance criteria are regularly tested to ensure that the quality, quantity and cost equation remains in balance.

Delegation

The ability to delegate is a crucial management competence facilitating the division of labour. It ranges from simple task-sharing to specialisation in rou-tine performance of the individual components of more complex operations.

Its appropriate application is essential to successful organisational growth but is limited by factors such as:

- the complexity of tasks entrusted to lower levels
- delegated responsibility and authority must be appropriate to the level of management
- the accountability of the delegate.

Below are a number of key points and tips to be considered.

Checklist of the guiding principles of delegation

▼   *Clarify relationships.* This is especially true where professional, functional or locational divisions in the organisation are already well-established practice. For example, confusion can easily arise in such complex organisations where in a multidisciplinary working situation persons of equal rank may not have similar delegated authority.

▼   *Make sure that delegation is at an appropriate organisational level.* Delegation of tasks, responsibility for whole tranches of work and/or appropriate decision-taking to other levels and spheres must be carefully judged to enhance performance. There are a number of sophisticated tests which can help assess exactly where this point should be. However, the limits are well recognised:

- too far or excessive delegtion causes self-perpetuating splinters and satellites with quasi-authority
- not far enough or too little delegation results in constant referrals for ratification of minor decisions.

▼   *Ensure that responsibility carries commensurate authority.* It is virtually impossible to successfully delegate responsibility without granting the necessary authority. If this quite common error is perpetuated in an organisation, it will lead to frustration and ultimately to failure.

▼   *Take care that managers who have delegated powers and responsibility are aware of their accountability.* Managers at all levels are sometimes unaware that the famous axiom 'delegation is not abdication' applies to them.

▼   *As far as possible maintain an open system of communications.* This means that the flow of non-confidential organisational information is not restricted to chains of command but is available on general release. Make every effort to release promptly organisational information that conforms with transparency.

Tips from the front office

▼ Arranging the transfer of powers, responsibilities and account-ability, and managing the outcomes can be costly.
▼ If there is more than one tier, for example in the public sector, these costs can escalate at an alarming rate.
▼ A balance has to be struck between the number and size of organisational strata and the cost incurred in simply managing them.

The delegation of spending powers to lower levels of an organisation implies hierarchical recognition of greater sophistication and complexity, and the acceptance that, in reality, the rate of resource consumption is determined by staff who are not accountants or members of the board. However, in budgetary management, it is important to truly reflect the needs of the organisation so that the delegation process is not simply geared to the cult of already powerful managers. The decision about where spending powers should be allocated must always be dependent on factors which limit the range, size and scope of production levels. Below are a number of key points and tips to be considered.

Checklist of points to be considered when delegating spending powers

▼ *Homogeneity*. Within potential budget management sites, similarities such as product or client groups, function, location, discipline or professionally linked staffing are the main considerations that identify a budget centre. However, it is not always possible to follow the same rule in each case. For example, within the same system, locational identifiers might be prevalent in some choices, whereas product or client groups might be deciding factors in others.
▼ *Budget size*. Budgets should be large enough to absorb reasonable fluctuations without creating a sense of crisis but should also be reflective of management realities.

  – Maximum delegation means more budget centres but much smaller budgets.
  – Selective delegated spending powers result in larger budgets and fewer budget managers.

- Optimum delegation happens where there is a regularity to budget sizes that produces the greatest flexibility.

Budget managers will wish to see the following key questions clarified in their budget agreements.

- What is the main objective workload?
- When is the objective to be achieved?
- How much is allocated for the task?
- What quality and quantity of resources can be purchased for this amount of money?
- What performance criteria will be used?

▼ *Viability* and manageability are key to the successful delegation of spending powers and the number of budget centres, together with any tiering that might occur, reflects these factors. The relationship between budget size and the total amount of money in a system can be expressed in the simplified equation

$$T - c = n \times b$$

where T is the total, c is the cost or the loss to the system due to overadministration, n is the number of proposed budget centres and b is the average size of a budget.

▼ *The potential budget manager.* Remember, potential budget managers will be drawn from departments that generate significant expenditure and will not often have financial backgrounds or business acumen. Therefore, clear and agreed objectives have to be set, together with the provision of training and expert support. Costs and benefits have to be taken into account and by applying the rules regarding homogeneity, size, viability, etc it is possible to arrive at the best choice (*see* Figure 7.1).

Tips from the front office

▼ Make compromises between maximum delegation and flexibility in order to produce a spending range which can be managed.
▼ Decide on initial rules for budget centres.
▼ Create a select list of potential budget centres and budget managers.
▼ Consider the cost and benefit of enhancing potential budget managers' competences.
▼ Revise acceptability criteria.

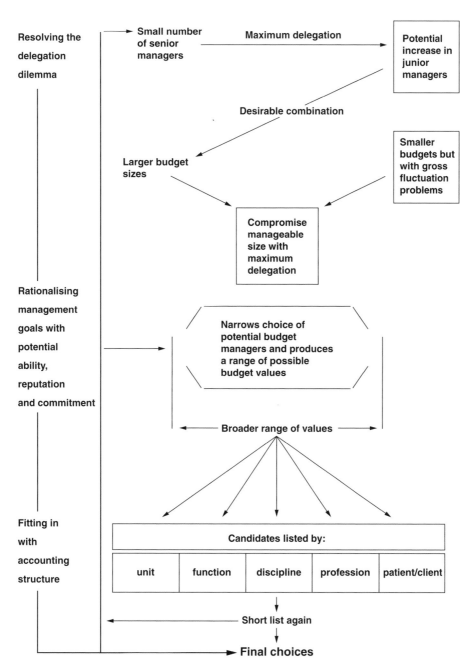

Figure 7.1   Budget manager selection process – considered rigidity spectrum illustrates the process and the considerations for the selection of a suitable budget management centre.

Organisational structure

Departmentalism

The following checklists cover the main considerations.

Checklist of division of labour

▼ It is in the nature of organisations to divide business into component parts so that a concentration of skilled effort can contribute to more beneficial outcomes.

▼ Most readers will be familiar with the concept of the production line in industry and will perhaps have heard of unfavourable comparisons with health and social care organisations.

Checklist of economies of scale

▼ The basic concepts inherent in specialisation and economies of scale underpin most cooperative efforts.

▼ In order to get the maximum benefit from scarce, specialised talents and other expensive resources, workloads tend to be concentrated into groupings, the largest being hospitals and the smallest community or social care teams.

▼ This conforms with the business management aim, which is to concentrate on discrete areas of activity.

▼ The rationale for the split into specialised divisions can be analysed according to the nature of the split: by profession, function or location.

▼ The most effective groupings within an organisational framework best follow the principles on which the organisation was originally constructed.

▼ This division has the advantage of using data which are common to all systems in such a way as to report the same overall position in different ways.

▼ Effective structure is therefore achieved through according entity status to each part and identifying the range of attributes which can readily be described and which will satisfactorily cover all structural options.

Entity

Entity is that attribute of a resource by which it is possible to assign it to a recognisable department. Broadly, an attribute describes:

- the identity of the resource, for example a social worker, a doctor or a piece of equipment
- where the entity is located, for example in the community, within a hospital ward or in an operating theatre
- the task that the resource performs, for example, services to the elderly, clinical services or general surgery
- its relationship to other similar items, for example, the department or budget to which the resource belongs.

If no rules were to be applied to limit the connection which each entity had with another, then every entity and its attributes would be treated in the same way. In other words, there would be no discernible structure. However, it is clear that organisational connections are both limited and enhanced by structure. The evolving organisational complexity significantly affects the structure because as rules are developed it is clear that other connections can be made which go beyond the attributes already developed. The simple choices are shown in the checklist below.

Checklist of choices for departmentalising

▼ *Entity grouping*
  - all entities form one whole budget
  - two budgets are created, one for people and one for all others
  - any other combination.

▼ *Functional grouping.* For example, cooks and provisions (catering); clerks and desks (administration); building and engineering (works and maintenance); doctors and nurses (clinical services); social workers, home helps, etc. (social services).

▼ *Relations groups.* The main professional groupings or disciplines, e.g. all domestic staff, clerical staff, furniture and estate, etc.

▼ *Locational groups.* Hospital site workers, resource centre, community, patch, etc.

▼ *Task groups.* Patients, clients, customers, etc.

▼ *Complex groups* which combine certain entity and attribute mixtures together for reasons other than those which are immediately apparent from Figure 7.1.

The degree and complexity of control can vary. An organisation's degree of sophistication in applying control factors will dictate its place on the spectrum. The main factors to be considered are whether the system is limited to:

- singular financial control
- financial control linked to specific resource purchasing power
- control, purchasing power and output measures linked in complexity
- outcome measures introduced to create composite data
- additional factors, etc.

As pieces of data are added to the selection model, two constraints are also introduced. The first is concerned with the timing of reporting and general communication. It is important that reports are both relevant and up to date. The more elements are added, the more likely it is that delays may occur. The second constraint concerns the possible impairment that might be caused to accuracy where the time factor is considered paramount.

The method of management control is itself another more subtle factor. With the model in its most simple form, reports may flow with almost complete freedom without any perceivable limitation. The implications of such an arrangement would be far reaching for an organisation because the economies of scale which are obtained from managing resources at a higher level are diminished as a result.

Structural shapes

If professional management is the model chosen, professional lines are secured at each level of the organisation in a vertical structure. This is illustrated in Figure 7.2.

This will produce strict departmental control at each level through professional lines but it causes difficulties when an attempt is made to become more flexible. For example, where a resource problem has been identified at Level 3 which requires a movement of resources from h1 to a1, the simplified string of communication would be:

$$h1 \rightarrow h \rightarrow h \rightarrow H \rightarrow \text{Executive board transfer} \rightarrow A \rightarrow a \rightarrow a \rightarrow a1$$

The delays, difficulties and cost to the decision-taking process at each level will result in the probability of inflexibility. However, there would be significant advantages in that this type of structure offers protection for each profession.

In practice, the structure of health and social care organisations is more flexible. They tend to be built on a mixture of divisional rules which favour the multidiciplinary approach. Thus a location such as a hospital site, a

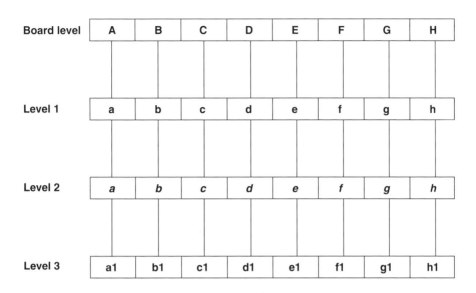

Figure 7.2   Division by profession.

residential home or a specialised unit might form the basis of department-alism. This is illustrated in Figure 7.3.

This model offers a great deal more flexibility in that the manager at each level can make decisions about the whole spectrum of activity. Although the communication string would be shortened, control is exercised at various levels to ensure that this is balanced with accountability. Thus each manager has clear responsibility and authority.

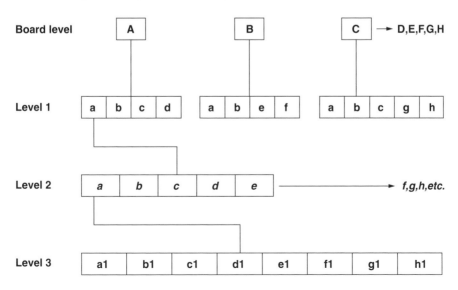

Figure 7.3   Flexible structure.

Most managers are aware that the creation of organisational momentum through innovation is a finite quantity because momentum is a constant. Innovative thinking is not the sole preserve of the boardroom. It is sometimes not long before conservatism and convention take hold. At best a conflict arises, at worst the desire to be creative is suppressed. Therefore, within the structure there must be devices whereby revolutionary aspects and ideas are neither diminished nor suppressed. In this context, it is worth reflecting on the influence that new and controversial thinking has had on past generations of managers and how it has come to affect our business philosophy today.

Budget profiles

Once the lines of communication have been agreed and clarified, and the organisational structure decided, the budget target can be calculated for each budget manager (zero, incrementalism, cost based, once-and-for-all projects or a combination of two or more). In order to simplify matters, budgets are of two principal types or a combination of them.

- Budgets to cope with recurring or day-to-day expenses such as payroll or monthly bills. The profile for recurring expenditure has to be spread over the total period, e.g. the financial year, or a month, etc. This means that some small variation in spending can be expected against a fixed target.
- Budgets to cover non-recurring expenses such as capital, refurbishment, or perhaps certain occasional payroll items such as overtime, sickness and holiday relief. Because they are termed non-recurring does not mean that the items will never occur again but rather that they don't happen regularly. This type of profile differs in that the amount of total budget added in each month is equal to the spend until the total amount of budget is exhausted. *At this point spending must cease.* In other words, the crucial measure of performance is not a variation from the target but continuous scrutiny of the balance remaining.

In the case of non-recurring budgets that are to be spent on more infrequent but often large-scale projects, e.g. replacement furniture or equipment, building and works contracts, or items that are entirely new, referred to as *capital equipment* or *capital works projects*, there is usually a considerable delay between the act of commissioning and the time when spending actually begins to occur.

- This is because the contract or order is placed some time before the items begin to be delivered or the work commences.
- Thus budget managers can be lulled into thinking they have more available funds than they actually have.

- In such cases, careful scrutiny of the commissioning process taken together with what is actually happening, is essential.
- Budget performance for *budgeted capital expenditure of £30k* over a 12-month period is illustrated in Figures 7.4 and 7.5 and in Table 7.1.

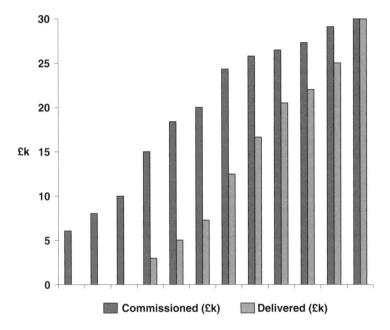

■ Commissioned (£k)   ■ Delivered (£k)

Figure 7.4   Illustration of £30k capital commissioning and delivery over a 12-month period.*

*Notes

- It can be seen that the commissioning process nearly reaches the target of £30,000 early in the year.
- However, deliveries came much later, starting slowly in July 2003.
- If, at the end of September 2003, the budget manager was not in possession of the complete picture, he or she might forecast total expenditure in the region of only £15,000.
- This shows how the project has to be kept under constant review.
- Adjustments have to be made as the year progresses.
- In this case, a review at December 2003 indicated that some of the orders would not be delivered and therefore other items were brought forward which did in fact conform to the time frame.
- The result is that the £30,000 budget was properly expended at the end of the financial year 2003/04.
- In creating a profile for this type of budget, it is only possible to examine the balance remaining at any time and to see what will actually be realistically delivered from those items that are still outstanding.

The actual detail of this is shown in Table 7.1. The links between each column are as follows:

● Items commissioned [column 1] minus those delivered [column 2] is equal to the amount outstanding [column 4].
● Total budget £30k minus amount commissioned [column 1] is equal to balance remaining [column 3], or column 1 plus column 3 is always equal to £30k.

Table 7.1   Illustration of 'balance remaining' principle

Commissioned (£k)	Delivered (£k)	Balance remaining	Outstanding
6	0	24	6
8	0	22	8
10	0	20	10
15	3	15	12
18	5	12	13
20	7	10	13
24	12	6	12
25	16	5	9
26	20	4	6
27	22	3	5
29	25	1	4
30	30	0	0

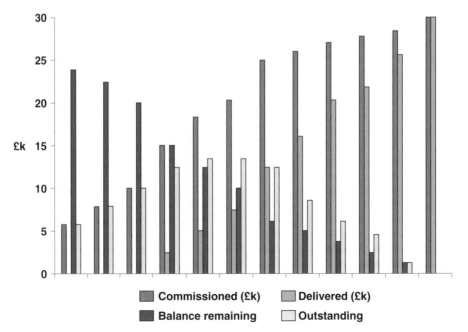

Figure 7.5   Balance remaining compared with outstanding orders.

Over the period of time involved, constant monitoring of the balance remaining together with the outstanding order position will have ensured that the budget was properly used. But it all depends upon reliable systems and good cooperation that link each part of the process. When commissioning reached the budget target of £30k then commissioning had to cease.

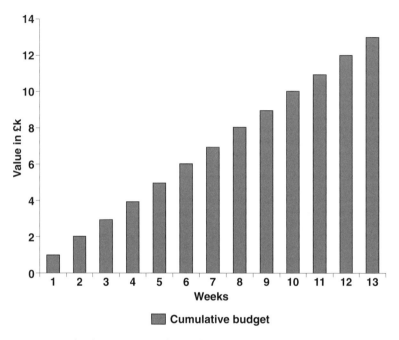

Cumulative budget

Figure 7.6 A perfectly even cumulative budget spend over a 13-week period.

However, because of variations and fluctuations in expenditure patterns, the perfection shown in Figure 7.6 is almost never achieved and to insist upon equal divisions would simply result in reports that were impossible to interpret without a large number of caveats.

Table 7.2 Simple budget profile

	Total budget (£)	July spend (£)	Cumulative to July (£)	Remainder (£)
Annual basic budget	1,200,000	100,000	400,000	800,000
Sickness and holidays	100,000	15,000	16,000	84,000
Overtime	57,000	5,000	19,000	38,000
Unsociable hours	64,000	5,100	20,300	43,700
Total annual budget	1,421,000	125,100	455,300	965,700

One of the most popular ways to deal with these types of variation and fluctuation is to take an estimated amount for each of the seasonal or workload pressures out of the basic annual budget. The basic budget can then be divided into equal segments for each time period and an amount added back in as the variable amounts are spent. An example of this type of calculation is shown in Table 7.2 on the previous page.

The profile shows the following points.

- Only £1,000 of the sickness and holiday contingency was used in the preceding three months, but the amount used in July was large. The budget manager would need to ensure that this was due to holiday demands and unlikely to continue.
- Although the cumulative position for overtime at the end of July seems reasonable, in fact, the July spend was £5k: if this rate continued, the forecast for the remainder of the year's spending would be 8 months @ £5k = £40k, which would mean that the year's budget would be overspent by £38k minus £59k (cumulative July spend £19k plus forecast for the rest of the year £40k). This equals an overspending of £21k. The budget manager therefore needs to make sure that the July spend is merely a seasonal fluctuation and will not continue at this rate.
- Unsociable hours payments are within budget.

Provided these matters are under the control of the budget manager, the overall trends and variations should be a reflection of the true position. The benefits of profiling are as follows.

- The resulting reduced basic budget should perform in a more consistent way.
- This will be more amenable to interpretation.
- Managers should be able to intervene with more confidence.
- Hopefully managers will be able to manage their budgets within the defined limits.

Case study

The 2004 summer holiday plan for weekly paid staff has been submitted to the director of clinical services at Smalltown Infirmary. A graphical representation is shown in Figure 7.7. Each member of staff will receive two weeks' holiday pay and the director has decided to 'borrow' the estimated extra cost from succeeding months. It has also been decided that additional temporary staff can be recruited from the sickness and holiday relief budget to cope with gaps in services such as portering, cleaning and housekeeping.

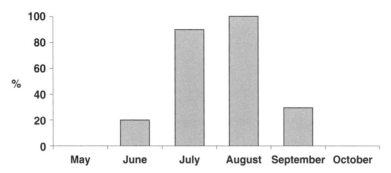

Figure 7.7 Holiday plan.

General points on contingency lists

Commissioners need to contemplate the necessity of additional expenditure because new services are constantly made available both through the development of medical and other technologies and through the improvements in best practice standards. They will therefore have a fairly consistent list of bids for new services and will maintain a contingency or other reserve to cope with these demands. In the joint project described in Chapter 6, p. 96, the amount held out was £1.7 million.

It would be unusual if the demands upon this money did not exceed the total amount available. The emerging picture could imply proposals for significant changes such as alterations to the balance of care, together with changes in the way resources are to be purchased, either direct from the market, rented, hired, subject to competitive tender, utilising the mixed economy of care, stimulating the voluntary sector, etc.

Proposed developments, interventions and retractions will have to be complemented by a range of various resourcing options. In the joint project described in Chapter 6, the joint project team reported on the likely savings to be made. Their calculations were the result of a detailed study, but in general the total savings amount plus other monies such as income equated with the idea of providing a more appropriate and seamless form of care for patients and clients in the defined categories. There would also be a saving of capital monies held in reserve.

Estimated long-term savings and sources of funding

* Direct revenue savings from Smalltown Infirmary
    ward closures   £550,000
* Expected income from patients/clients   £200,000
* Savings from rationalisation within St Bediful's Hospital   £200,000
                                                                    ‾‾‾‾‾‾‾‾
                                                                    £950,000

Table 7.3   Estimated cost of developments

Outline of developments	Current year (£k)	Full year (£k)
High dependency unit		
● developing, extending and enhancing staffing levels	100	110
Day surgery facilities and dedicated staffing		
● improvements in facilities and increased staffing	100	150
● extension of day procedures, having due regard to the appropriateness, recovery time needed, fitness for discharge and domestic arrangements	250	520
Accident and emergency		
● improved staffing levels and facilities	100	100
General acute services		
● waiting list initiative and significant increases in medical and nursing staff numbers	160	300
Care of the older patient		
● selected pilot schemes for the introduction and evaluation of pathways of care	*	120*
● development of differentiated response to care management considering the greatly increased levels of demand	140	280
● capital cost of structural alterations, incorporating compliance with building standards, and refurbishment of the 'new' ward block at Smalltown Infirmary	500*	
Rehabilitation		
● reshaping health and social care to promote greater independence for patients and clients (daily living)	*	120*
Bridging finance	350	
Totals	1700	1700
Repayment of bridging finance		350
Net totals	1700	1350

*These figures indicate the areas where duplication has taken place. Although the amounts are not now counted twice, there still remains the possibility of further negotiation over their future because the joint project plan clearly indicates that it is more than self-balancing. The commissioner might therefore reallocate them to other more pressing demands.

Thus in the case of the joint project, this list includes a number of items that are applicable to the initiative proposed by the joint project team. On the developmental side, bids for additional funding to support the balance of care initiative were still being considered, but initial estimates were as follows.

- Capital cost of refurbishing and commissioning the 'new' ward block at Smalltown Infirmary to accommodate assessment and rehabilitation unit, and to include day hospital and respite day centre – £500,000.
- Revenue cost of care of patients/clients – £560,000.
- Revenue cost of day hospital and rehabilitation facilities (daily living, etc.) – £120,000.
- Additional revenue costs of a multidisciplinary pathway of care team for individual assessment and care management to cover short, medium and longer-term needs, including acute and after care – £57,000.
- Additional cost of comprehensive rehabilitation and follow-up programmes to enable individuals to make the transition towards greater independence – £47,000.
- Additional cost of arrangements for management development, monitoring, review and evaluation of programmes – £50,000.

In the business plan proposals, which in the longer term are almost self-financing, there is a need for interim bridging finance in order to facilitate the development. The amounts are shown opposite in Table 7.3.

Intervention

Where there are significant variations it will be necessary to intervene or to reallocate. Effective intervention depends on reliable and timely information on performance. Interventions are of two types – strategic and tactical. Strategic intervention, like rationalisation for example, takes longer to activate and will be reserved for longer-term gains. Tactics are used on a daily basis but must be applied within the overall strategy of the organisation, for example specific service reductions where it was explicity intended to expand that particular service. The checklist below provides details of the most common forms of intervention.

Checklist of budget intervention strategy and tactics

▼   *Waste*. This is a resource manager's ongoing obligation, but drive on waste can be enhanced by using process quality (*see Managing Health and Social Care: essential checklists for frontline staff*).[1]

▼ *Delay*. Options for delay in the purchasing and commissioning of new or replacement resources have to be considered in the contexts set out in Chapters 5 and 6.

▼ *Increase*. Where a significant underspending is predicted, managers often increase the rate of expenditure on appropriate resources. This has the effect of mopping up any excess funds.

▼ *Moritorium*. Sometimes it is appropriate to call a temporary halt to staff recruitment or other commitments such as overtime. This gives time and space to a resource manager wishing to review their operation. However, where there are pressing contractual obligations, resource levels have already been defined and this option is therefore negated.

▼ *Reductions*. In certain circumstances, a manager may decide to reduce staffing or other resource levels, for example where efficiency can be increased using mechanical means.

▼ *Workloads*. In contractual situations, managers may decide to reduce workloads to contract levels (*see* Chapter 4). In appropriate circumstances it might be more efficient to increase workloads, for example where an increase may cause the average cost to fall. Generally speaking though, in situations where workloads have fallen to near zero, managers will have to take a decision as to the overall future of that particular service.

▼ *Value for money commissioning and purchasing*. Improved performance in the domain of purchasing and commissioning will produce longer-term savings.

▼ *Rationalise*. In the climate of change a rationalisation of a service is always a distinct possibility and managers must be prepared for this type of situation.

▼ *Retract*. A retraction in service provision may sometimes be expedited by developments elsewhere either on the technical or clinical front or with alternative forms of care and treatment. This would be a strategic issue and needs to be considered in the broadest possible sense.

▼ *Close or stop*. In extreme cases where funds have been exhausted, it may be that certain projects can be halted without detriment to the immediate future of the service, for example painting programmes.

▼ *Increase budget*. A redirection or reallocation of funds is always an option where there has been a clear case of underfunding and, of course, where funds are available.

▼ *Strategic alliances*. A budget manager may enter a strategic alliance or partnership in appropriate circumstances in order to obtain the best use of resources and to provide a better, more seamless service (*see* Chapters 1 and 8).

▼ *Obtain alternative.* It may be possible to obtain alternative forms of help or funding (*see* Chapters 1 and 8).
▼ *Consider early retirement* and write memoirs exposing the inequities of the system!

Tips from the front office

▼ At the beginning of the financial year, carefully check the way your new budget has been calculated.
▼ Ensure that you know what is being charged to your budget and that you have commissioned or authorised the purchase of all personnel and items. In particular, frequently check the names on the payroll and make sure that they can be reconciled with actual people you know are within your span of control.
▼ If you had a consistent underspending in the previous period and no contrary actions occurred in the meantime, you will expect to find the same trends reflected in the current period.
▼ A contradictory overspend indicates that there has been a mistake in the calculations.
▼ Now is the time to sort it out! Don't delay!
▼ Check out all the elements that are contributing to cost. For example, do you receive internal services from another budget manager in the Central/local Sterile Supply Department (CSSD), laundry, catering, stores, pharmacy, maintenance, etc?
▼ What are all these charges?
▼ Do you sign for them without checking even the basic requisitions? Do you check the items when they are received?
▼ Are you ordering or accepting too much? What would happen if you stopped ordering them or accepting them?
▼ Look over your spending policies. Are you conforming with official stationery, postage and telephone usage, and energy policies?
▼ What about those payroll extras such as overtime, etc? Are they out of control? If you don't know, take advice.

Key action points

▼ Budgets and budget statements must be accurate indicators of financial performance.

▼ They must arrive in time and clearly show the need for appropriate intervention.

▼ Two-way communication is essential to successful budgetary management.

▼ The budget structure must reflect clearly the lines of management responsibility and authority.

▼ Delegation of spending powers has to include authority as well as responsibility.

▼ Budgets have to be viable – large enough to absorb day-to-day fluctuations, but small enough to be capable of delegation.

▼ Methodologies used for budget setting must be fit for the purpose and clearly reflect objectives.

▼ Budget contents, i.e. the items or personnel to be commissioned, purchased or employed must be under the control of the manager and be clearly related to the workload focus or centre of activity.

▼ Budget profiles must be appropriate and calculated to reflect changing patterns.

▼ Contingency plans must be adequate.

Case study

St Bedeful's Chief Executive had strategic concerns relating to the introduction of foundation hospitals, the GP contract and the possible closure of Smalltown Infirmary casualty department.

- A nearby hospital had gained foundation status and there was the possibility that key staff would be attracted away.
- St Bedeful's accident and emergency department already had increasing numbers of patients waiting on trollys for considerable lengths of time. Investigations revealed that this was due in part to difficulties experienced by patients who needed a GP at night or at the weekend and who now came straight to casualty.

Closure of Smalltown casualty department would have a significant impact on St Bedeful's already overstretched resources.

Reference

1   Bryans W (2004) *Managing Health and Social Care: essential checklists for frontline staff*. Radcliffe Medical Press, Oxford.

8

Managing in the political dimension

The acquisition and consumption of resources are not in themselves objectives, but are rather the means by which objectives can be obtained. However, a manager's ability to influence the main funding provider and to compensate for shortfalls by using suitable alternatives is an important asset in sustaining and developing services. In addition, managers must create an internal environment that attracts the right calibre of staff. Resource managers must also be able to implement their plans. This chapter examines the framework that will enhance these capabilities.

The issues

- Managers have to clearly identify and distinguish between their internal and external environments.
- They must value, develop and sustain all those sources that may be of use to them in maintaining and improving their services.
- Managers must become skilled at managing their external environment (the political dimension).
- They must deliberately plan to foster relations with

  - local supporters (voluntary workers, charities and media management)
  - main resource sources, including connections with labour and supplies markets
  - other statutory authorities, national charities and private enterprise.

- Managers need to underpin these endeavours with sound internal relations. Where appropriate, external arrangements should be made more formal by developing partnerships.

Introduction

Health and social care political dimensions are complex interactions between individual managers and other participants, who directly or indirectly affect the environment in which a particular manager operates and functions. In order to manage within these contexts, managers have to have both a vision of the way in which they must proceed and an understanding of the main factors that will influence their success.

As far as all organisations are concerned, the need for increasingly sophisticated arrangements due to more and more intense specialisation results in a greater degree of dependence and interdependence based on reliable departments. If their performance is satisfactory, many of these departments will be mostly invisible, particularly those that provide a service such as payroll. Others, especially those that have a more dramatic impact, will have a high profile. Thus a culture can easily be allowed to grow that encourages the notion that if it's invisible, then that portion of the organisation can sustain a greater slice of 'the hard times'.

In resource management, a manager's main purpose is to attract good quality resources for consumption within their boundaries that have the most beneficial effect on their patients/clients. This means complete comprehension of *all* those goods and services that are used internally. In return, managers have to provide value added services to their external environment. No matter where managers are placed within an organisation, whether they are devoted to direct patient/client care and are therefore well away from the 'business side' or whether they work within one of the more hotel-oriented parts of an organisation, they all act as both consumers and providers.

Similarly, whether managers are engaged in either the commissioner or provider mode, as far as their own departments are concerned, they still conform to these apparently anomalous roles. This definition, which is a paradox based on the commissioning/providing processes, applies equally well to the paymaster as it does to the clinical or social care manager. The checklist below is a reminder of some of the key coterminous managers whose services may form some of the resources that cross another budget manager's boundary (a clinical or social care manager in this example).

Checklist of coterminous managers

▼   *Hotel and infrastructure*
     – building or estate services
     – catering contract manager

  - cleaning/portering contractor
  - transport services
  - laundry contractor.

▼ *Business services*
  - payroll and related services
  - supplies/stores/logistics management
  - human resources/personnel managers
  - accounts and invoices
  - finance managers.

▼ *Related clinical or paramedical services*
  - pharmacy
  - laboratories
  - radiology
  - paramedical managers
  - Central/local Sterile Supply Departmental requirements (CSSD), etc.

This paradox is illustrated in Figure 8.1 overleaf.

Funding problems

As stated earlier, an increase in funding is not necessarily the key to service improvement or development. Indeed additional money for a specific purpose may not in itself remedy deficiencies in other facets of resource management. It will not facilitate the purchase of other scare resources where no such resources exist. In other words, the money will remain unspent. Generally, this is often the situation with human resources. Not many health or social care organisations have a full complement and if they achieve their targets, they often cannot retain that position for long. Where such circumstances are to a large extent prevalent, it does not make good financial sense to leave that money in place until such time as all vacancies are filled.

Conversely, funding shortages often occur apparently at random and are due in part to costs exceeding the money that is available. However, sometimes shortages may be due to a change in the funding rules where a less favourable means of allocation has been agreed. The new national tariff for certain procedures is one example, another is the change in the grant system for local authorities.

Thus when we speak of a funding crisis, we may be referring to either under or overfunding. Unfortunately, in health and social care organisational

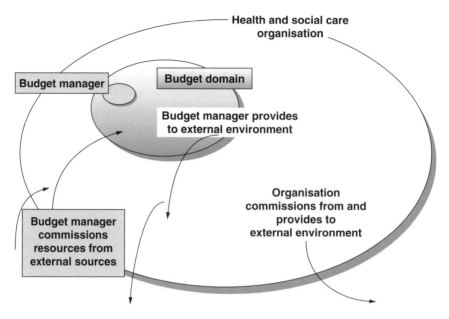

Figure 8.1   Commissioning paradox.*

*Notes
- A budget manager is usually one of many in an organisation.
- As a corporate body, all these managers acting together make up the totality of the organisation and therefore affect their individual and overall performance.
- All budget managers are interdependent.
- Across individual boundaries, they transact many items of business.
- This is sometimes called 'quasi-trading'.
- Whether they are engaged as commissioners or providers, they commission appropriate resources for internal consumption and provide value-added services to their external environment.
- At some previously determined level, a flow of funds has to underpin these arrangements. For example, the levels chosen for money flowing inwards might be calculated per case, case mix or block allocation. Money flowing outwards may be determined according to an individual contract (a pay packet) or by any other measurable means that can be verified later.
- It is of significant interest that, contrary to popular opinion, payments outwards in respect of resources received are well defined and subject to fairly rigorous checks, whereas the flow of funds coming into health and social care is connected to specific services provided within less well-defined limits that in the event of a crisis or in the case of anomalies cannot truly be controlled.
- There is therefore a tendency among commissioners of health and social care to exploit this situation because in a crisis providers have to make immediate responses.

culture, the inevitably pessimistic expectation is a frequent reality. So how do we know that there is a funding crisis? Below is a checklist of the most common sources of intelligence.

Checklist of funding crisis information sources

▼   *Reliable source.* Occasionally a resource manager may be casually informed by a member of the management team before any official announcement.
▼   *Budget statements.* These should be the most reliable source of crisis information and should pre-empt any rumours.
▼   *Guess work.* Experienced resource managers can often read the signs of crisis before they occur.
▼   *Rumours.* Office or departmental gossip is often the basis of reality.
▼   *Previous experience.* Resource managers may know from experience that there will be a crisis in the funding at specific times in the year and this may be compensated later when matters are brought under control.
▼   *Discover it yourself.* A resource manager may become suddenly aware from their own records and indications that untoward events are about to precipitate a crisis, for example the discovery that a building is unsafe.

Despite the allocation of funds that are to be spent on specific purposes, most managers have an instinctive drive to accomplish tasks with less effort, thus creating savings or surpluses. Indeed, the demand for the achievement of more quality activity for less money (QUALM) is a phenomenon common to both health and social care.

However, this phenomenon may be prevalent to an unreasonable extent in the upper reaches of an organisation, characterised by constant cuts based on the assumption that 'they can do what they did last year'. As we shall see, this is a blunt instrument in a sophisticated world. Unfortunately it also generates the growth of a disparate contrary subculture which encourages waste by creating demands for more than is needed (DEMN).

But what are savings or surpluses? Are they, for example, the end products of all those hundreds of efforts to reduce costs that are made daily by diligently cost-conscious managers? Do we mean the development of better working practices, probably using more modern techniques and technology? Are they the results of major initiatives that involve restructuring, rationalisation and retraction?

Influencing the external environment

In order to compensate for the constant scarcity experienced, resource managers need to become competent in managing the external environment. Below is a 'map' of how this complex activity can be fitted together.

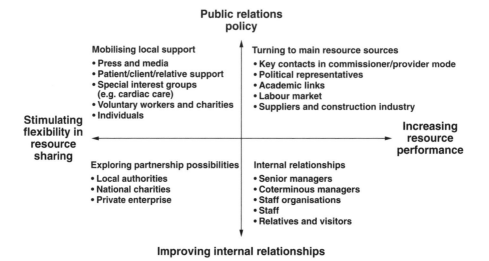

Figure 8.2 Outline map of main external environmental contacts.

Checklist of main business considerations

▼ Apart from the obvious management considerations, the definition of a boundary that separates a budget manager's domain from the external environment is important because of the real and quasi-trading activities that are transacted within the overall organisational framework, i.e. between one department and another and on behalf of the organisation as a whole.

▼ Although budget managers' performance in the internal environment is subject to well-established measures, their record of managing their external environment is not so well regulated or documented.

▼ The continued provision of value-added goods and services to their external environment is dependent upon reciprocal funding or help in kind.

▼ They must therefore develop competences that enable them to manage these external pressures better.

▼ Figure 8.2 opposite illustrates the main outline of the contacts that need to be fostered to achieve this particular management function.

▼ This will be a focus for budget managers who wish to develop further their competences in managing their external environment.

▼ Below are a series of further checklists that will stimulate managers to review the ways in which they might improve their external relations and develop strategic partnerships or alliances that have beneficial consequences for the partners.

Checklist of criteria for choice of partners or allies

▼ *Definition of specific problem areas.* The problem areas need to be coterminous, for example, between health and social care organisations where a seamless service for designated patients/clients can be arranged.

▼ *Compatible objectives.* Joint objectives must conform to the culture and ethos of both prospective partners.

▼ *Size and scope of the problem* need to be significant for formal arrangement to be put in place. In other words, the process must be worthwhile so that shared resources produce savings that can be spent inwardly, for example reducing duplication of effort.

▼ *Willing and appropriate partners.* There must be a cooperative spirit which motivates joint action and will not generate internal opposition.

▼ *Expectation of improved outcomes.* The arrangement should have clear benefits for clients and patients, for example the provision of appropriate forms of care at suitable levels.

▼ *Setting objectives.* The arrangement must indicate how objectives are set and have reporting mechanisms put in place that are acceptable.

▼ *Implementation process and management.* There must be a clearly defined and agreed process for implementation so that all objectives are achieved.

▼ *Organisation and management development.* With the new emphasis on cooperation and revised reporting structures, management development must be made compatible with organisational development. Staff must understand and sign up to the revised arrangements.

▼ *Evaluation.* An agreed system for the evaluation of performance at all levels needs to be in place and where further changes seem necessary, a system of revision agreed.

Checklist of benefits to be derived from partnerships with other statutory providers

▼   Development of the so called 'seamless service' for service users whose needs transcend perceived boundaries of statutory responsibility, for example care of the older patient and child protection.
▼   Singularity and clarity in the budget context will be more efficient and effective.
▼   Improve the harmony and alignment of existing organisational cultures.
▼   Help develop a unitary approach to service provision.
▼   Provide multidisciplinary management and staff development to inculcate a consistent sense of purpose.
▼   Make previously intractable problems more amenable to solutions, for example patients and clients receiving excessive levels of care and treatment that unnecessarily tie up valuable resources.
▼   Create a situation where existing resources can be better utilised and where additional resources may be more accessible and available.
▼   Stimulate creative and innovative attitudes.

Checklist of general considerations where alliances are to be made with other sources, for example with a supplier

▼   *Specific considerations*

External influences
  – Legality. Make sure that the proposal does not infringe the law.
  – Ethics. Check that there is no conflict of interest nor damage to integrity (everyone is aware of the smoking habit/tobacco industry connection but there are many other more subtle factors).
  – Equity. Test whether the proposal is targeted on an individual or group within an organisation.
  – Intention. Be certain that the proposed alliance does not provide an external provider with an unfair advantage, for example in a separate contract situation.

Internal constraints
  – Appropriateness. A proposal must be appropriate to the strategic requirements of the organisation.

- Revenue consequences. Where there is a sharing of expensive equipment (e.g. scanners), there will be ongoing costs and these must be carefully considered before proceeding.
- Utility and obsolescence. The proposal must have a realistic utility for the organisation.

▼   *Coordination.* A designated senior manager or director should have responsibility for coordinating various interests, for example clinical considerations, public relations, supply chain management, finance or total quality management.

▼   *Communication and review.* This must be undertaken by both or all parties.

Communicating with the external environment

The fundamental challenge inherent in the management of change, particularly where it involves further scarcity, lies in the alleviation and reduction in the concern levels felt by staff, clients, patients and the public about the services and structures with which they have become familiar. This involves a number of tractable complications which can be diminished or avoided altogether.

Checklist of tractable complications

▼   *Ultra vires rules.* It is essential that authority is not exceeded, so that a trust, individual or other body cannot be discovered to be in breach of or acting beyond their powers, for example the use of private property or endowment and gift funds for purposes other than those designated.

▼   *Reliability of the database.* Fact-gathering and the establishment of acceptable reference points are essential to the success of any project, for example the disproof of clinical statistics.

▼   *Exhaustion of all areas of research and opinion.* The exploration of all shades of opinion and their discount, if that is appropriate, must be exhaustive so that it can be shown that every possible alternative was examined.

▼   *Litigious censure.* The abuse of any of the above can result in or be the foundation of legal action.

▼ *Judicial review*. There have been a number of applications in this context based on the alleged inadequacy of the consultative process. Often the application for a review is rejected on the grounds that there is no legal right to consultation and failure to grant it in the form and depth required is not an entitlement because of 'procedural impropriety.' It is important therefore to ensure that the correct procedure is applied at all times and in all cases.

There are a number of key points to bear in mind.

Checklist of key points on communications

▼ Determination of a general communications policy that embraces key quality standards such as the fostering of an atmosphere of openness and honesty.
▼ Recognition that communication is not one way. This means making people feel *really* involved – taking time with them, listening, debating, making notes and *suiting them* if possible.
▼ Development of a public relations strategy that makes information freely available through convenient and timely devices.
▼ Preparation of information for, and later, consultation with patient and client representations and pressure groups or other related organisations.
▼ Consultation with staff groups, trades unions, staff associations, consultative committees and professional bodies through established channels for their involvement in service changes.

Although some setbacks can be expected, there are a few key principles on quality that must be incorporated into external dealings.

Checklist of communication objectives

▼ Creating a climate of awareness.
▼ Ensuring the communication process is effective (i.e. setting measurement criteria and applying them).
▼ Designating a consistent focal point where information can be obtained. This means that the same person or department gives both the good news and the bad news. There is no policy of

selection. This is crucial to credibility, but it also means making sure that that person is well briefed.

▼ Designing a freedom and availability of *accurate* information that is *full* enough for ordinary people to feel they can judge.

▼ Informing and convincing everybody about the proposed improvements.

▼ Making people feel valued and that they will be heard.

Checklist of public relations initiatives

▼ Seminars or blaster sessions to introduce the concepts and topics which have influenced the proposed changes.

▼ Short briefings by the management board or directors involved in the business planning process for health councils, etc.

▼ Face-to-face meetings with officers from trades unions.

▼ Meetings with affected staff groups. However, make sure that these do not contravene any agreements with trades unions relating to the general consultative process.

▼ Regular management information bulletins or house journals.

▼ Leaflets covering the particular area of interest.

▼ Mobile exhibitions incorporating all relevant items of interest.

▼ Tape and slide packages to support any of the above facets.

▼ Regular issue of press releases.

▼ Specific briefing sessions for journalists and editors (maybe regular contact).

▼ Meetings covering all relevant external bodies.

▼ Offering specialised speakers to community groups, schools, etc.

▼ Open days to cement trust and cooperation.

▼ Design and development of websites.

Tips from the front office

▼ Speak out early.

▼ Be truthful.

▼ Give people time to organise opposition.

▼ Engage those 'Save our …' groups in proper dialogue.

Human resources

In an uncertain climate, the possibilities for industrial unrest are legion. Staff and staff organisations naturally feel frustrated and threatened. They will react to belated information in a hostile and unhelpful way. It is vital that managers at all levels strenuously seek to avoid any unnecessary anxiety. This means they must all participate in a positive consultative process that both gives and takes information. A human resource strategy, developed specifically to be sensitive in this vital resource area, is therefore essential.

Tips from the front office

▼ Make sure you know the attitude, policy and consultative arrangements of your organisation.
▼ Ensure that you fully comprehend how it supports the management of change.
▼ Ask whether it is consistent with service-wide principles and practice.

The human resource agenda for the management of change should include the following issues.

Checklist of principles guiding human resource communications

▼ The determination to maintain equity and equality at all change junctures.
▼ Recognition of the essential nature of developing partnership and collaborative structures with trades unions and professional organisations.
▼ There must be agreement on the precise circumstances for internal trawl and/or more open competition for specific vacancies.
▼ The observation and implementation of development, deployment and other reallocation arrangements arising out of established good practice and centred on the cadre of existing staff who have contributed to and are affected by the new structural arrangements.

Checklist of human resource key issues

▼ Production of management and staff development initiatives to encourage and sharpen existing staff skills for the interim and longer-term stages of the business planning project.
▼ Development of agreed arrangements for the slotting in of existing staff to posts of commensurate responsibility and conditions, where competition would be wasteful and overly disruptive.
▼ Internal or external competition arrangements and the circumstances where these are clearly necessary.
▼ The application of agreed re-deployment rules within the organisation.
▼ Arrangements for the protection of pay and conditions.
▼ Agreed redundancy policy for handling selection, offers and acceptance criteria.
▼ Agreement on the way to handle the complaints of staff who may feel aggrieved at their treatment following the rearrangement of posts and jobs. It is important to identify areas which will be recognised as giving reasonable grounds for appeal and a procedure agreed by which they can be equitably heard.
▼ Application of termination payments for senior managers and for variations in terms and conditions where, for example a merger is contemplated.

Key action points

▼ Managers must define their internal and external environments and increase their competence to manage and influence external forces.
▼ They have to balance opportunities with resources.
▼ Managers have to create a direction so that they can develop services.
▼ All alternative resource sources must be explored and exploited in order to maintain and improve services.
▼ They must develop communication skills and strategies that will support service development and change, and these must work internally and externally.
▼ They must become politically astute.

▼   They must take steps to create a seamless service that bridges the gaps in service provision that currently cause inappropriate and expensive blockages at critical points.

▼   Resource managers want to develop partnerships that will enhance the quality of service delivery within their commissioning area.

Postscript

Case studies

- Mr H O'Condriac has been elected chairman of the Bigtown Patients' Forum and has been appointed Honorary Governor of St Bediful's. In these dual roles, he is waging a crusade to improve cleanliness and believes that catering, cleaning and portering services should be brought back under the direct control of health and social care managers. He is indifferent to the cost and other resource implications of withdrawing from existing contracts. He is also convinced that short-stay patients, unless there are good medical grounds, should be given food that they would normally receive at home.

- The joint project involving St Bediful's, Smalltown Infirmary and Bigtown Social Services promises to provide more suitable cost-effective alternatives to unnecessary hospital stays, care-home arrangements and other expensive forms of care packages. And it will increase independence for physically disabled people through rehabilitation and a more integrated approach by means of clinical, therapeutic, social and environmental interventions. However, for strategic reasons it has been decided to abandon the idea of locating the unit in Smalltown Infirmary and to place it in the old sanatorium building, which is part of the St Bediful's Hospital complex. It has been renamed 'The Near-Home Facility' and has been refurbished and developed at a lower estimated cost to better facilitate the discharge of elderly patients/clients from one level of care and admit them to another lower and more appropriate form without the need to rush patients or clients into making life-changing decisions about their future. Operating through appropriate teams it will be managed on a strict short-term stay policy. It will also provide accommodation for respite care.

- At Smalltown Infirmary, due to persistent key staff shortages, the Accident and Emergency Department has been closed indefinitely. This, in addition to the loss of the promised refurbished wards, has caused dismay and the local papers are unanimously backing a 'save our hospital campaign'.

Useful websites

- www.doh.gov.uk/finman
- www.doh.gov.uk/waitingtimes
- www.hm-treasury.gov.uk
- www.dpp.org.uk
- www.auditcommission.gov.uk
- www.communitycare.co.uk
- www.integratedcarenetwork.gov.uk
- www.kingsfund.org.uk

Recommended reading

- Bryans W (2004) *Managing in Health and Social Care: essential checklists for frontline staff.* Radcliffe Medical Press.
- Stewart R (2002) *Evidence Based Management.* Radcliffe Medical Press.
- Glasby J (2003) *Hospital Discharge: integrating health and social care.* Radcliffe Medical Press.
- Phillips A (2002) *The Business Planning Toolkit.* Radcliffe Medical Press.
- Peck E (2005) *Organisational Development in Healthcare.* Radcliffe Publishing.
- Semple Piggot C (2000) *Business Planning for Healthcare Management.* Open University Press.
- Moulin M (2002) *Delivering Excellence in Health and Social Care.* Open University Press.
- Maxwell R (1984) Quality assessment in health. *BMJ.* **13**: 31–4.
- Walshe K (2003) *Regulating Healthcare: a prescription for improvement?* Open University Press.
- McDonald R (2002) *Using Health Economics in Health Services: rationing rationality?* Open University Press.
- Codling S (1998) *Benchmarking.* Gower.
- Hyde J and Cooper F (eds) (2001) *Managing the Business of Health Care.* Harcourt Health Sciences/RCN.
- Baxter C (ed.) (2001) *Managing Diversity and Inequality in Health Care.* Harcourt Health Sciences/RCN.
- Young A and Cooke M (eds) (2001) *Managing and Implementing Decisions in Health Care.* Harcourt Health Sciences/RCN.
- Glasby J and Littlechild R (2004) *The Health and Social Care Divide: the experience of older people.* The Policy Press.
- Leathard A (ed.) (2003) *Interprofessional Collaboration: from policy to practice in health and social care.* Routledge.

Index

Page numbers in *italics* refer to tables or figures.